Evolving Therapies in Esophageal Carcinoma

Editor

WAYNE L. HOFSTETTER

THORACIC SURGERY CLINICS

www.thoracic.theclinics.com

Consulting Editor
M. BLAIR MARSHALL

November 2013 • Volume 23 • Number 4

ELSEVIER

1600 John F. Kennedy Boulevard • Suite 1800 • Philadelphia, Pennsylvania, 19103-2899

http://www.theclinics.com

THORACIC SURGERY CLINICS Volume 23, Number 4
November 2013 ISSN 1547-4127, ISBN-13: 978-0-323-24237-0

Editor: Jessica McCool
Developmental Editor: Susan Showalter

Thoracic Surgery Clinics (ISSN 1547-4127) is published quarterly by Elsevier Inc., 360 Park Avenue South, New York, NY 10010-1710. Months of publication are February, May, August, and November. Business and editorial offices: 1600 John F. Kennedy Boulevard, Suite 1800, Philadelphia, PA 19103-2899. Periodicals postage paid at New York, NY, and additional mailing offices. Subscription prices are $350.00 per year (US individuals), $453.00 per year (US institutions), $165.00 per year (US Students), $435.00 per year (Canadian individuals), $585.00 per year (Canadian institutions), $225.00 per year (Canadian and foreign students), $465.00 per year (foreign individuals), and $585.00 per year (foreign institutions). Foreign air speed delivery is included in all Clinics' subscription prices. All prices are subject to change without notice. **POSTMASTER:** Send address changes to Thoracic Surgery Clinics, Elsevier Health Sciences Division, Subscription Customer Service, 3251 Riverport Lane, Maryland Heights, MO 63043. **Customer Service (orders, claims, online, change of address): Telephone: 1-800-654-2452 (U.S. and Canada); 314-447-8871 (outside U.S. and Canada). Fax: 314-447-8029. Email: journalscustomerservice-usa@elsevier.com (for print support); journalsonlinesupport-usa@elsevier.com (for online support).**

Reprints. For copies of 100 or more, of articles in this publication, please contact Commercial Rights Department, Elsevier Inc., 360 Park Avenue South, New York, NY 10010-1710. Tel: 212-633-3874; Fax: 212-633-3820; E-mail: reprints@elsevier.com.

Thoracic Surgery Clinics is covered in *MEDLINE/PubMed (Index Medicus), EMBASE/Excerpta Medica, Science Citation Index Expanded (SciSearch®), Journal Citation Reports/Science Edition,* and *Current Contents®/Clinical Medicine.*

Printed and bound by CPI Group (UK) Ltd, Croydon, CR0 4YY

Transferred to digital print 2012

Contributors

CONSULTING EDITOR

M. BLAIR MARSHALL
Associate Professor of Surgery, Georgetown
University School of Medicine; Chief, Division
of Thoracic Surgery, Department of Surgery,
Georgetown University Medical Center,
Washington, DC

EDITOR

WAYNE L. HOFSTETTER, MD
Professor of Surgery and Director of Esophageal
Surgery, Department of Thoracic and
Cardiovascular Surgery, The University of Texas
MD Anderson Cancer Center, Houston, Texas

AUTHORS

JAFFER A. AJANI, MD
Professor of Medicine, Department of
Gastrointestinal Medical Oncology, The
University of Texas MD Anderson Cancer
Center, Houston, Texas

NASSER ALTORKI, MD
Professor of Cardiothoracic Surgery and Chief,
Division of Thoracic Surgery, Department of
Cardiothoracic Surgery, New York
Presbyterian Hospital, Weill Cornell Medical
College, New York, New York

EUGENE H. BLACKSTONE, MD
Professor of Surgery, Cleveland Clinic Lerner
College of Medicine of Case Western Reserve
University; The Kenneth Gee and Paula Shaw,
PhD, Chair in Heart Research, Department of
Thoracic and Cardiovascular Surgery, Heart
and Vascular Institute, Cleveland Clinic,
Cleveland, Ohio

MARIELA A. BLUM, MD
Assistant Professor of Medicine, Department
of Gastrointestinal Medical Oncology, The
University of Texas MD Anderson Cancer
Center, Houston, Texas

ARTUR BODNAR, MD
Department of Thoracic Surgery and Thoracic
Oncology, Virginia Mason Medical Center,
Seattle, Washington

GAIL E. DARLING, MD, FRCSC, FACS
Director of Clinical Research in Thoracic
Surgery, Toronto General Hospital, Royal
College Chair Thoracic Surgery Specialty
Committee, Professor of Thoracic Surgery,
Kress Family Chair in Esophageal Cancer,
Department of Surgery, University Heath
Network, University of Toronto, Toronto,
Ontario, Canada

MARTA L. DAVILA, MD
Professor of Medicine, Department of
Gastroenterology, Hepatology and Nutrition,
and Associate Director, Cancer Prevention,
The University of Texas MD Anderson Cancer
Center, Houston, Texas

WAYNE L. HOFSTETTER, MD
Professor of Surgery and Director of Esophageal
Surgery, Department of Thoracic and
Cardiovascular Surgery, The University of Texas
MD Anderson Cancer Center, Houston, Texas

TOSHITAKA HOPPO, MD, PhD
Department of Surgery, Institute for the Treatment of Esophageal and Thoracic Disease, The Western Pennsylvania Hospital, Allegheny Health Network, Pittsburgh, Pennsylvania

DAVID H. ILSON, MD, PhD
Gastrointestinal Oncology Service, Department of Medicine, Memorial Sloan-Kettering Cancer Center, New York, New York

BLAIR A. JOBE, MD, FACS
Chief, Department of Surgery; Director, Institute for the Treatment of Esophageal and Thoracic Disease, The Western Pennsylvania Hospital, Allegheny Health Network, Pittsburgh, Pennsylvania

MARK J. KRASNA, MD
Medical Director, Meridian Cancer Care, Neptune; Clinical Professor of Surgery, Rutgers Robert Wood Johnson Medical School, New Brunswick, New Jersey

GEOFFREY Y. KU, MD
Gastrointestinal Oncology Service, Department of Medicine, Memorial Sloan-Kettering Cancer Center, New York, New York

DONALD E. LOW, FACS, FRCS(C)
Head of Thoracic Surgery and Thoracic Oncology, Virginia Mason Medical Center, Seattle, Washington

JENIFER MARKS, MD
Division of Thoracic Surgery, Hackensack University Medical Center, Hackensack, New Jersey

SUBROTO PAUL, MD
Assistant Professor of Cardiothoracic Surgery, Division of Thoracic Surgery, Department of Cardiothoracic Surgery, New York Presbyterian Hospital, Weill Cornell Medical College, New York, New York

DAVID C. RICE, MD
Associate Professor, Department of Thoracic and Cardiovascular Surgery, The University of Texas MD Anderson Cancer Center, Houston, Texas

THOMAS W. RICE, MD
Professor of Surgery, Cleveland Clinic Lerner College of Medicine of Case Western Reserve University; The Daniel and Karen Lee Endowed Chair in Thoracic Surgery, Department of Thoracic and Cardiovascular Surgery, Heart and Vascular Institute, Cleveland Clinic, Cleveland, Ohio

NABIL RIZK, MD
Department of Surgery, Thoracic Service, Memorial Sloan-Kettering Cancer Center, New York, New York

HEATH D. SKINNER, MD, PhD
Assistant Professor of Radiation Oncology, The University of Texas MD Anderson Cancer Center, Houston, Texas

B. MARK SMITHERS, MBBS, FRACS, FRCSEng, FRCSEd
Associate Professor, Director, Upper GI, Soft Tissue Unit, Princess Alexandra Hospital, The University of Queensland, Buranda, Brisbane, Australia

KAZUKI SUDO, MD
Post-doctoral fellow, Department of Gastrointestinal Medical Oncology, The University of Texas MD Anderson Cancer Center, Houston, Texas

STEPHEN G. SWISHER, MD
Chair, Department of Thoracic and Cardiovascular Surgery, The University of Texas MD Anderson Cancer Center, Houston, Texas

TAKASHI TAKETA, MD
Post-doctoral fellow, Department of Gastrointestinal Medical Oncology, The University of Texas MD Anderson Cancer Center, Houston, Texas

IAIN THOMSON, MBBS, FRACS
Upper GI, Soft Tissue Unit, Discipline of Surgery, Princess Alexandra Hospital, The University of Queensland, Buranda, Brisbane, Australia

ROOPMA WADHWA, MD
Post-doctoral fellow, Department of Gastrointestinal Medical Oncology, The University of Texas MD Anderson Cancer Center, Houston, Texas

Contents

Radiographic and Endosonographic Staging in Esophageal Cancer 453

Mark J. Krasna

Radiographic imaging using computed tomographic (CT) scan and positron emission tomography/CT are primarily helpful in identifying distant metastases. In general, if patients have evidence of lymph node involvement that is proved pathologically by endoscopic ultrasound/fine needle aspiration, this information is considered definitive, and the patient can be referred for the appropriate stage-specific therapy. Laparoscopy combined with laparoscopic ultrasound and peritoneal lavage has been shown to have sensitivity of 67% and specificity of 92% for lymph node disease. Thoracoscopy may help identify involved lymph node in the mediastinum before resection and help determine the field of radiation.

Esophageal Cancer Staging: Past, Present, and Future 461

Thomas W. Rice and Eugene H. Blackstone

TNM cancer staging, conceived 70 years ago, was first applied to the esophagus in 1977. Prior staging was neither data-driven nor harmonized with stomach cancer. Machine-learning analysis of worldwide data addressed these shortcomings in the 7th edition. The 8th edition considers 6 problems in attempting to advance esophageal cancer staging.

Personalizing Therapy for Esophageal Cancer Patients 471

Toshitaka Hoppo and Blair A. Jobe

Management of esophageal cancer starts with accurate tissue diagnosis and clinical staging. Advances in screening and surveillance programs and endoscopic techniques have resulted in patients with early-stage esophageal cancer diagnosed more frequently. Endoscopic mucosal resection for staging is essential to diagnose T1a cancer and crucial to exclude risk factors for progression to cancer or presence of concomitant cancer. Esophagectomy is an essential component of treatment of locally advanced, resectable esophageal cancer. Despite intensive multidisciplinary approaches, the prognosis of esophageal cancer is unacceptable. This article focuses on the process of decision making used to select optimal therapy for esophageal cancer.

Endoscopic Management of Barrett's Esophagus with High-Grade Dysplasia and Early-Stage Esophageal Adenocarcinoma 479

Marta L. Davila and Wayne L. Hofstetter

Several endoscopic procedures have been recently developed for the treatment of Barrett's esophagus and early esophageal cancer, including endoscopic resection, radiofrequency ablation, and cryoablation. This review article discusses ideal candidates for endoscopic therapies, current treatment modalities, clinical and safety outcomes, and specific management recommendations.

Determining what defines an adequate esophageal resection to optimize long-term outcomes in esophageal cancer is an elusive goal. The primary reason for this ambiguousness is the almost total lack of good quality prospective randomized surgical trials that examine this question adequately. Most available data are derived from small retrospective series typically representing single institution series and their treatment biases. The intent of this article is to identify the goals of an appropriate esophagectomy for cancer, essentially defining the targets that should be achieved from an operation.

Despite advances in treatment, long-term outcomes for esophageal cancer remain poor, with overall survival rates of between 15% and 35%. Poor long-term survival reflects locoregionally advanced disease or metastatic disease at presentation. Among patients undergoing surgical resection, 40% to 50% have stage III disease. Surgery alone results in poor locoregional control and poor long-term outcomes, with survival rates ranging from 10% to 30%. Induction therapy combining surgery with chemotherapy with or without radiotherapy attempts to improve long-term survival in these patients. This article examines the merits of various modalities of induction therapy for patients with locally advanced esophageal cancer.

In patients with operable esophageal cancer, there is evidence supporting the use of preoperative chemotherapy or preoperative chemoradiation. The addition of radiotherapy to chemotherapy seems more relevant for the more locally advanced cancers. There is a need to examine in trials more modern chemotherapy combinations with and without concurrent radiation and for research into assessing methods for predicting outcomes from neoadjuvant therapy as part of the paradigm of therapy for this disease.

This article focuses on adjuvant (postoperative) strategies for locally advanced esophageal cancers. Results of completed phase III trials of postoperative therapy for locally advanced adenocarcinomas and squamous cell carcinomas (SCCs) of the esophagus and gastroesophageal (GE) junction are summarized. Several postoperative and perioperative strategies have been shown to improve survival by approximately 15% when compared with surgery alone for adenocarcinomas of the esophagus and GE junction. On the other hand, all proven strategies for resectable SCCs involve preoperative treatment, and there are no validated strategies for the postoperative treatment of SCC.

THORACIC SURGERY CLINICS

Preface
Evolving Therapies in Esophageal Carcinoma

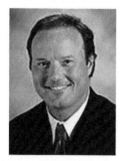

Wayne L. Hofstetter, MD
Editor

The landscape of esophageal cancer therapy has changed significantly over the past decade. Whereas surgery had historically been the only therapy that could offer a reasonable opportunity for cure, we have entered an era where there are multiple treatment pathways that may lead to a favorable result from therapy. What brought us to such a point? Disruptive technologies are frequently borne from unmet need. Surgery remains the ultimate therapy to achieve local and regional control of disease, but unfortunately, not every patient is amenable to the radical extirpative surgery that is required to achieve these excellent results. Some do not have the physiologic capability to withstand surgery, while others have disease that is either too advanced or too early to be optimally treated by major resection: an under- or overkill phenomenon. Enter in, alternative treatment algorithms.

I am fortunate to have trained under brilliant mentors with a deep understanding of esophageal cancer. From them I learned the creativity and capability of good esophageal surgery. And, I also learned about the limitations. The nature of esophageal cancer puts the clinician and patient at a distinct disadvantage; most patients present in an advanced stage of disease. Our overall goal is to expand the subset of patients that are potentially curable rather than merely super-selecting the population that may be amenable to current therapies. We need to devise and adopt methods of treatment that expand on the capabilities of

surgery to improve overall survival for the whole population. Unfortunately many of our current treatment algorithms redundantly emphasize local-regional disease and lack significant efficacy at the systemic level. We still have a long way to go with systemic and induction therapy for esophageal cancer. Missing from this issue is a discussion on emerging therapies and biomarker research. At this time, these avenues of research are promising to exploit genetic mutation for therapy and guide treatment based on tumor response. My hope is that by the next time *Thoracic Surgery Clinics* is ready to revisit esophageal cancer therapy that there will have been significant advances in these areas to report on.

I am indebted to the contributing authors, whose work is presented in this collection of articles emphasizing a multimodality perspective on esophageal cancer care. I thoroughly enjoyed reading each and every manuscript and I learned from every author. There are some very unique concepts presented here, including the goals for future staging systems, international agreement on complications reporting, and quality-of-life research that should affect the way we consider and offer therapy. The reader will notice some similarity of the combined modality topics from article to article, but each author provides a unique and interesting perspective on the current options for treatment ranging from early to locally advanced cancers. It is vital that we as surgeons understand the data and direction of clinical research for

Thorac Surg Clin 23 (2013) ix–x
http://dx.doi.org/10.1016/j.thorsurg.2013.08.002
1547-4127/13/$ – see front matter © 2013 Elsevier Inc. All rights reserved.

adjunctive and nonsurgical treatment options for esophageal cancer. In many cases, surgeons can and should be directly involved even when the therapy does not specifically call for resection.

Finally, I would like to offer thanks to Mark Ferguson, who would not take no for an answer and encouraged me to take on this issue, to Blair Marshall for seeing this project to fruition, and most of all, to Jessica McCool, whose pleasant reminders kept this issue moving forward in the face of mounting deadlines and delays. I hope that you all enjoy reading this issue as much as I have.

Wayne L. Hofstetter, MD
The University of Texas, MD Anderson
Cancer Center
1515 Holcombe Boulevard, Unit 445
Houston, TX 77030-4009, USA

E-mail address:
whofstetter@mdanderson.org

Radiographic and Endosonographic Staging in Esophageal Cancer

Mark J. Krasna, MD[a,b],*

KEYWORDS

- Esophageal cancer • Staging • Imaging • Radiographic staging • Esophageal ultrasound

KEY POINTS

- Staging is crucial to appropriate therapy of esophageal cancer.
- Radiographic imaging is primarily helpful in identifying distant metastases.
- Endoscopic ultrasound (EUS) and EUS/fine-needle aspiration are crucial to determining respectability and extent of locoregional disease.
- Modern staging using computed tomography and positron emission tomography can identify metastatic disease as well as predict response to therapy.

INTRODUCTION

Staging of esophageal cancer is critical to determining optimal therapy in all patients with this disease. Current use of multimodality therapy in these patients requires a clear understanding of the stage at the time of presentation. This understanding allows us to avoid unnecessary treatment in patients with limited, local disease as well as allows those patients with metastatic disease to receive appropriate treatment and palliation as soon as possible.

ROLE OF STAGING

Current staging systems depend primarily on the depth of invasion in the wall, the presence of lymph nodes involved with tumor, and the identification of distant metastatic disease.[1] The allocation of tumor-node-metastasis (TNM) stage-to-stage groupings is determined by survival; this has been confirmed by the report from the World Esophageal Cancer Consortium, which documented the relationship between staging and survival.[2] The order of testing should allow

the treating physicians to arrive at the decision regarding whether definitive treatment is feasible as quickly as possible (**Box 1**).[1,3]

The most common presenting signs of squamous cell carcinoma or locally advanced adenocarcinoma are dysphagia and odynophagia. For patients with Barrett esophagus and early-stage adenocarcinoma, reflux is the most common presenting sign. Severe weight loss usually occurs after swallowing difficulties begin. Upper esophageal tumors can involve the recurrent laryngeal nerve, causing the patient to have a hoarse voice. Phrenic nerve involvement can trigger hiccups. A postprandial or paroxysmal cough may indicate the presence of an esophagotracheal or esophagobronchial fistula resulting from local invasion by a tumor.[4,5]

Radiography and upper endoscopy are the most important investigations for evaluating the presence of and extent of esophageal cancer. If esophageal cancer is suspected, the first investigation is usually an upper gastrointestinal endoscopy (esophagogastroduodenoscopy). This endoscopy allows assessment of any obstruction and biopsy to confirm the histology of mucosal

Disclosures: The author has nothing to disclose.
[a] Meridian Cancer Care, 1945 Route 33-Ackerman South, Room 553, Neptune, NJ 07753, USA; [b] Rutgers-Robert Wood Johnson Medical School, 125 Paterson Street, New Brunswick, NJ 08903, USA
* Meridian Cancer Care, 1945 Route 33-Ackerman South, Room 553, Neptune, NJ 07753, USA.
E-mail address: MKrasna@meridianhealth.com

Thorac Surg Clin 23 (2013) 453–460
http://dx.doi.org/10.1016/j.thorsurg.2013.07.002
1547-4127/13/$ – see front matter © 2013 Elsevier Inc. All rights reserved.

Box 1
TNM classifications

Grade

GX: Grade cannot be assessed

G1: Well differentiated

G2: Moderately differentiated

G3: Poorly differentiated

G4: Undifferentiated

Primary Tumor (T)

TX: Primary tumor cannot be assessed

T0: No evidence of primary tumor

Tis: High-grade dysplasia

T1a: Tumor invading lamina propria or muscularis mucosae

T1b: Tumor invading submucosa

T2: Tumor invading muscularis propria

T3: Tumor invading adventitia

T4a: Tumor invading pleura, pericardium, or diaphragm

T4b: Tumor invading other adjacent structures

Regional Lymph Nodes (N)

NX: Regional lymph nodes cannot be assessed

N0: No regional lymph node metastasis

N1: Regional lymph node metastasis involving 1–2 nodes[a]

N2: Regional lymph node metastasis involving 3–6 nodes[a]

N3: Regional lymph node metastasis involving 7 or more nodes[a]

[a] Regional lymph nodes extend from periesophageal cervical to celiac nodes.

Distant Metastasis (M)

MX: Distant metastasis cannot be assessed

M0: No distant metastasis

M1: Nonregional lymph node metastasis or distant metastasis

Stage

Stage 0: T0 N0 M0, any grade; Tis N0 M0, any grade

Stage IA: T1 N0 M0, grade 1–2

Stage IB: T1 N0 M0, grade 3; T1 N0 M0, grade 4; T2 N0 M0, grade 1–2

Stage IIA: T2 N0 M0, grade 3–4

Stage IIB: T3 N0 M0; T0 N1 M0, any grade; T1–2 N1 M0, any grade

Stage IIIA: T0–2 N2 M0, any grade; T3 N1 M0, any grade; T4a N0 M0, any grade

Stage IIIB: T3 N2 M0, any grade

Stage IIIC: T4a N1–2 M0, any grade; T4b any N M0, any grade; any T N3 M0, any grade

Stage IV: any T, any N, M1, any grade

---

lesions.[6] Confocal laser endoscopy with targeted biopsy can improve the diagnostic yield for neoplasia and decrease the number of mucosal biopsies in patients in the surveillance group. Endoscopy can identify benign causes of obstructive symptoms as well as allow an opportunity for dilatation and immediate palliation.[7]

RADIOGRAPHIC DIAGNOSIS AND STAGING

A barium swallow is sometimes done before endoscopy to confirm an obstruction, but this is not routinely required. Barium swallow was used in the past as a tool to identify esophageal cancer before endoscopy. Although it can provide information on tumor length, features such as location and size of the tumor are more accurately assessed by endoscopy. Barium studies cannot accurately rule out benign disease or rule in malignancy without a biopsy and are therefore of little value as an initial diagnostic test, unless one is suspicious of a tracheoesophageal fistula. They may provide supportive data in the differentiation of gastroesophageal junction tumors from gastric tumors where large tumors are seen on retroflexion.[8]

Computed tomography (CT) is still the gold standard for *staging* patients identified with esophageal cancer. This primarily allows the identification of distant metastatic disease in the lungs, abdominal viscera, and bones. In the absence of metastatic disease, CT can provide some idea of local invasiveness as a guide to determining local resectability. In specific, CT can detect contact with the airway or major blood vessels, which might be an indication of unresectability.[9]

CT scan of the chest and abdomen is performed if the suspicion of esophageal cancer is high or biopsy confirms the diagnosis. The CT scan assesses tumor bulk and can monitor tumor response to therapy. The CT can define whether the tumor has spread from the esophagus to regional lymph nodes and/or contiguous structures. Oral and intravenous contrast material should be used to ensure optimal pacification of the lumen and visualization of the heart, mediastinal vessels, and liver. An esophageal wall thickness greater than 5 mm is abnormal suggesting a T2 or higher lesion. T1 and T2 lesions generally show an esophageal mass thickness between 5 mm and 15 mm; T3 lesions show a thickness greater than 15 mm. T4 lesions show invasion of contiguous structures on CT and may be suspected by the presence of "contact" between the esophagus and surrounding structures, such as the airway or great vessels. In general, contact with the aorta of more than 90° circumference is considered suspicious for T4 disease.[10] In addition, diaphragmatic invasion is suggested by loss of the retrocrural fat planes. Tracheal invasion may be suspected where a midesophageal tumor bulges into the posterior membranous portion of the airway. Suspicious contact with the airway should be followed-up with bronchoscopy. CT has relative limitations for identification of regional nodal metastases. Its use depends on size criteria; lymph nodes greater than 1 cm in short-axis are considered suspicious for malignancy. Of course smaller lymph nodes are also frequently involved, and larger lymph nodes may simply be reactive.[9] Visceral metastases to the lungs, bone, and liver are most common and most easily suspected by CT. Many metastases are readily detectable by CT (sensitivity 81%). The evaluation of the lung fields to identify pulmonary metastases is best performed by high-resolution contrast-enhanced CT scan. CT has relatively poor specificity (82%) and cannot readily differentiate between indeterminate pulmonary nodules and metastatic disease. Many esophageal cancer metastases are occult or are difficult to prospectively diagnose by CT alone. CT scan reassessment of response to therapy has sensitivity for persistent disease of only between 27% and 55% and a specificity of 50% to 91% partially due to difficulty differentiating residual cancer and reactive inflammation.

Magnetic resonance imaging (MRI), in general, has not panned out as advantageous over CT or other imaging techniques. With the advent of PET scanning, MRI does not appear to hold an advantage for detection of unsuspected metastatic disease. Some early reports did suggest that MRI was better in determining local invasion to the airway or vessels, but this has not met with wide acceptance. MRI is highly accurate for detecting distant metastases, especially to the liver and adrenals, and for determining advanced local spread (T4). However, it is less reliable in defining early infiltration (T1 to T3). MRI appears to be sensitive in predicting mediastinal invasion; the loss of signal in the vessels and the air-filled trachea and bronchi may provide a clear delineation between the tumor and the aorta and the tracheobronchial tree. Like CT scans, MRI scans also tend to understage the regional lymph nodes.

A recent review of the world's literature determined that in the near future MRI has the potential to bring improvement in staging, tumor delineation, and real-time guidance for radiation therapy and assessment of treatment response.[11] Although historically poor, recent improvements in MRI protocols and techniques have resulted in better imaging quality and the valuable addition of functional information. Similar or even better results have been achieved using optimized MRI compared with other imaging strategies for T-staging and N-staging. Recent pilot studies showed that functional MRI might be capable of predicting pathologic response to treatment and patient prognosis.

Positron emission tomography (18F)-fluoro-2-deoxy-D-glucose positron emission tomography (FDG-PET) scanning can now identify anatomic lesions that have significant suspicion on functional imaging to be malignant; this has not obviated the need for biopsy, however, as false-positive results on PET are known to occur. Suspicious lesions should generally still be confirmed by histologic diagnosis to avoid over-diagnosis of metastatic disease, which may lead to a patient receiving inadequate therapy. Given the importance of identifying distant disease, PET should be performed early on in the process of staging. Our current approach is to perform CT imaging once the diagnosis of esophageal cancer is made. This is then followed by PET/CT before EUS or other evaluation of resectability. Use of PET improves the accuracy of staging and facilitates selection of patients for surgery, by detecting distant metastatic disease not identified by CT alone. PET has a higher sensitivity than CT for detecting nodal and distant metastases and a higher accuracy for determining resectability than CT. FDG-PET also has limitations in determining regional disease because "spill-over" signal from an adjacent primary tumor may render detection of regional nodes difficult. This is otherwise known as a Halo-effect. A small locoregional nodal or visceral metastases (<8 mm) may not be reliably identified by current PET technology. Overall, PET is recommended to improve the accuracy of M-status for the staging work-up of patients with esophageal cancer who are potential candidates for curative therapy.[12–19]

Although FDG avidity in the esophagus is suspicious for primary tumor, this may also occur secondary to esophagitis, previous interventions, and mucosal ulceration. Therefore, evaluation of the apparent metabolic activity of the primary esophageal tumor should be correlated with pathologic findings at endoscopy. PET may also help identify occult submucosal disease, which is important in treatment planning.

RESTAGING WITH PET

Another potential use of PET is for the detection of responses to chemotherapy and radiation therapy. FDG-PET imaging can identify changes in glucose uptake, which may be a better indicator of a favorable response to treatment when compared with anatomic changes seen on other imaging studies such as CT scan. Data from the MUNICON study as well as from MD Anderson have shown the potential value of PET scan as a restaging tool. This tool is primarily useful after neoadjuvant induction chemotherapy followed by chemoradiation and then surgery. In this setting, it can be used as a means of identifying patients who are not candidates for resection because they develop distant metastasis early on. Likewise, if a patient does not respond to induction chemotherapy, they are unlikely to benefit from continuing chemoradiation with the same agent but rather should consider either going directly to surgery or continuing with an alternative regimen of chemotherapy with the radiation.[20]

The report of the MUNICON 2 trial and the upcoming results of MUNICON 3 should establish the role of PET in restaging patients with esophageal cancer undergoing induction therapy.[21] Because of insufficient evidence, no specific recommendation has been made for or against the use of PET for the assessment of treatment response and the evaluation of suspected recurrence until the recent report of The Society of Thoracic Surgeons Guidelines (**Box 2**). Relative changes in FDG-uptake of esophageal cancer are better prognosticators. Early metabolic changes from pretreatment PET to post-treatment PET may provide the same accuracy for prediction of treatment outcome as late changes from PET to PET. PET has value in the assessment of neoadjuvant therapy response in patients with esophageal cancer. A 50% reduction in standardized uptake value (SUV) between pretherapy and post-therapy PET scans performed in the first 2 weeks after the initiation of neoadjuvant chemotherapy is the optimal condition for predicting a response to neoadjuvant therapy in patients with esophageal cancer.

After completion of any neoadjuvant therapy, restaging results in a patient being categorized as either having a complete response, a partial response, progressive disease or no response. Patients can also simply be assigned a new clinical stage identification based on the restaging results. Post-induction therapy stage is identified by the "y" prefix before the new clinical stage TNM designation (eg, yc TxNxMx). PET/CT scans are superior for identifying residual disease with a

sensitivity of 32% and specificity of 90%. Erasmus and colleagues found false-positive results with sensitivity of 43% and specificity of 50%, which was probably caused by chemoradiation-induced ulceration. PET scans may also spare some patients futile operations by finding new, interval distant metastases. Patients whose PET scan SUV decreased more than 50% after chemoradiotherapy had a longer overall survival and lower risk of death following surgery. Municon II identified 50 metabolic responders (decrease in SUV of more than 35%) who did not reach their median overall survival at 2 years after surgery as opposed to 54 nonresponders who had a median survival of 35.8 mos ($P = .002$). Klaeser and colleagues[22–24] found a limited predictive value of PET scans for response; sensitivity was 68% and specificity 52% with a positive predictive value of 58% and a negative predictive value of 63%.

ENDOSCOPIC ULTRASOUND

Once a tissue diagnosis is made, endoscopic ultrasound (EUS) is performed immediately after a PET/CT shows no evidence of metastatic disease. EUS is one of the newer modalities used in the staging of esophageal cancer, although stenosis can limit its use. In addition, lymph nodes at a distance of more than 2 cm from the esophageal lumen cannot be imaged because of the very limited penetration depth of ultrasound. EUS can help in assessing whether a tumor can be resected or not. Findings that indicate unresectability include invasion into the left atrium; the wall of the descending aorta, spinal body, pulmonary vein, or artery; or tracheobronchial system. Especially in patients with disease of the middle and upper thirds of the esophagus, bronchoscopy with biopsy, fine-needle aspiration (FNA), or brushings can be helpful in determining involvement of the tracheobronchial tree. FNA can be performed into mucosal lesions within the lumen or transbronchially into lesions adjacent to the airway. EUS has become a standard in the workup for patients with esophageal cancer and should not be left out, especially in the context of a clinical trial and when considering surgery.[20]

EUS/FNA

Complete staging is now possible with EUS-FNA sampling of regional lymph node using a cytology needle. If this gives positive result, the need for thoracosocpy or laparoscopy is obviated. EUS can also be performed with ultrasound-guided needle biopsies through the EUS endoscope. Currently, EUS combined with FNA is the most

---

Box 2
NCCN and STS guidelines for diagnosis and staging esophageal cancer

Guidelines

The recent Society of Thoracic Surgeons/American Association for Thoracic Surgery guidelines from the taskforce on esophageal cancer define several steps along the diagnostic path for esophageal cancer with evidence to support their inclusion in an algorithm. Listed here are the recent guidelines recommendations excerpted with their level of evidence:

Diagnostic Guidelines

NCCN clinical practice guidelines in oncology: esophageal and esophagogastric junction cancers (excluding the proximal 5 cm of the stomach). Published by: National Comprehensive Cancer Network Last published: 2011[3]

Summary: This guideline provides a comprehensive overview of the diagnostic approach for this cancer.

Esophageal cancer: clinical practice guidelines for diagnosis, treatment, and follow-up.

1. The diagnosis should be made from an endoscopic biopsy, with the histology to be given according to the WHO criteria. Small cell carcinomas must be identified and separated from squamous cell carcinomas and adenocarcinomas, and be treated accordingly.

2. Staging should include clinical examination, blood counts, liver and renal function tests, endoscopy (including upper aerodigestive tract endoscopy in case of squamous cell carcinoma), and a CT scan of the chest and abdomen. In candidates for surgical resection, esophagogram and endoscopic ultrasound have to be added to evaluate the T (and N) stage of the tumor, and to assist in the planning of the surgical procedure. When available, PET may be helpful to identify otherwise undetected distant metastases or in diagnosis of suspected recurrence.

3. In locally advanced (T3/T4) adenocarcinomas of the esophagogastric junction infiltrating the anatomic cardia, laparoscopy can rule out peritoneal metastases.

4. For selection of local treatments, the tumors should be assigned to the cervical, intrathoracic esophagus or to the esophagogastric junction. The stage is to be given according to the tumor-node-metastasis system, with corresponding American Joint Committee on Cancer stage grouping.

STS Workforce on Esophageal Cancer

Class I Recommendation: For early-stage esophageal cancer, CT of the chest and abdomen is an optional test for staging (Level of Evidence B).

Class I Recommendation: For locoregionalized esophageal cancer, CT of the chest and abdomen is a recommended test for staging (Level of Evidence B).

Class IIB Recommendation: For early-stage esophageal cancer, PET is an optional test for staging (Level of Evidence B).

Class I Recommendation: For locoregionalized esophageal cancer, PET is a recommended test for staging (Level of Evidence B).

Class IIA Recommendation: In the absence of metastatic disease, endosonography (EUS) is recommended to improve the accuracy of clinical staging (Level of Evidence B).

Class IIA Recommendation: Endoscopic Mucosal Resection (EMR) should be considered for small, discrete nodules or areas of dysplasia when the disease appears limited to the mucosa or submucosa as assessed by EUS (Level of Evidence B).

Class IIB Recommendation: In locally advanced (T3/T4) adenocarcinoma of the esophagogastric junction infiltrating the anatomic cardia, or Siewart type III Esophagogastric tumors, laparoscopy is recommended to improve the accuracy of staging (Level of Evidence C).

Restaging (STS Taskforce)

Class I Recommendation: Restaging studies following neoadjuvant therapy before resection are recommended to rule out distant metastatic disease (Level of Evidence B)

Class IIA Recommendation: EUS restaging for residual local (mural) disease is inaccurate and can be omitted (Level of Evidence B)

Class IIA Recommendation: PET scan is recommended after neoadjuvant therapy for restaging to detect distant metastatic disease (Level of Evidence B).

accurate imaging modality for locoregional staging of esophageal cancer. EUS is close to 90% accurate in predicting initial T-stage before treatment, and assessment of N-stage is between 38% and 73% accuracy. FNA of lymph node can be expected to increase the accuracy further. These results are observer dependent and clearly improve over time with experience. Given the high specificity and low level of false-negative results, EUS is particularly good for its negative predictive value.[25–28]

Interpreting EUS findings after neoadjuvant therapy is similarly challenging and this procedure frequently overstages patients. Inflammatory changes associated with response are indistinguishable from persistent disease; specifically, the alternating sonographic bright and dark layers are obliterated by both viable tumor and scar related to a therapeutic response. Yen and colleagues investigated the efficacy of EUS for restaging esophageal cancer after neoadjuvant therapy and found the sensitivity to be only 5% and the specificity to be 38%. Eloubeidi and colleagues[29] assessed the true negative rate of EUS-FNA in 107 patients and found a specificity of 88% and a negative predictive value of 78%.[30]

Although EUS is extremely accurate for staging untreated esophageal cancer, its accuracy in staging tumors after neoadjuvant chemoradiation is relatively poor, with most errors due to overstaging. Accuracy of T staging falls to between 27% and 82% if used after neoadjuvant therapy. Errors in post-therapy staging are likely due to the similar echogenic appearance of fibrosis and residual tumor. Residual nodal disease is an ominous finding. EUS combined with FNA is very useful in detecting residual cancer within lymph nodes and may play a future role in selecting patients after neoadjuvant therapy who should be candidates for resection.[31]

ENDOSCOPIC MUCOSAL RESECTION

Endoscopic mucosal resection (EMR) has emerged as an important tool, primarily for patients with early-stage esophageal cancer. In this setting, an EMR can result either in an adequate resection of a T1a tumor or as a staging technique to augment EUS as a way of defining tumor depth. A positive margin after EMR requires a further, deeper surgical resection.[32] Specific guidelines for use of EMR as a staging tool have not yet been proliferated. The indications, conduct, and interpretation of results from EMR will be more fully discussed in subsequent articles.

THORACOSCOPY AND LAPAROSCOPY

If the EUS/FNA shows no lymph node involvement, thoracoscopy and laparoscopy are still generally used as definitive staging tools and have been used to help accurately stage patients before treatment. In one study, routine laparoscopy in 369 patients with esophageal cancer noted intra-abdominal metastases in 14% and celiac lymph node metastases in 9.7%. Laparoscopy combined with laparoscopic ultrasound and peritoneal lavage has been shown to have sensitivity of 67% and specificity of 92% for lymph node disease.[33] CT, MRI, and EUS can guide surgeons to focus on suspicious areas to maximize yield. This approach can provide greater accuracy in the evaluation of regional and celiac lymph nodes. This information is very important in patient

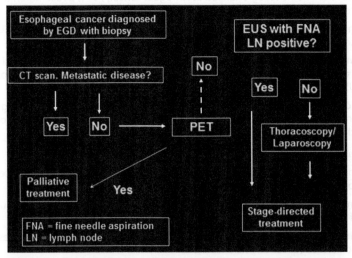

Fig. 1. Algorithm for evaluation and staging of esophageal cancer.

stratification and selection of therapy, especially in the setting of new treatment protocols. Furthermore, the histologic status of mediastinal and abdominal lymph nodes is critical for the design of the field for irradiation. It allows for maximizing dose delivery to areas of known disease, while minimizing dose to surrounding sensitive, normal tissue. Several reports have indicated the value of routine laparoscopic peritoneal washing and cytology in patients with esophageal and gastric adenocarcinoma.[34–38]

OTHER RADIOGRAPHIC TESTS

Chest radiograph has a minimal role in the modern diagnosis and staging of esophageal cancer, although it can reveal an abnormal finding in almost half of patients with esophageal cancer. However, in some countries, chest radiograph is still used routinely to identify hilar or mediastinal adenopathy, evidence of pulmonary metastases, secondary pulmonary infiltrates caused by aspiration, and pleural effusion.

Barium swallow is still used by some physicians to determine the length of involvement of an esophageal cancer. This has generally been supplemented by endoscopy and EUS as these are done routinely to obtain a tissue diagnosis and can determine not only the degree of mucosal wall invasion but also submucosal spread better than any radiographic tests.

Although abdominal ultrasound and liver scans are still used occassionally in some countries, their value is exceeded by the use of PET/CT and are only of historical significance.

SUMMARY

Staging is crucial to appropriate therapy of esophageal cancer (**Fig. 1**). Radiographic imaging is primarily helpful in identifying distant metastases. EUS and EUS/FNA are crucial to determining respectability and extent of locoregional disease. Modern staging using CT and PET can identify metastatic disease as well as predict response to therapy. Patients who have evidence of lymph node involvement, which is proved pathologically by EUS/FNA, can be referred for the appropriate stage-specific therapy. These evidences have been used to help accurately stage patients before treatment. Thoracoscopy/laparoscopy combined with laparoscopic ultrasound and peritoneal lavage has been shown to have high sensitivity and specificity for lymph node disease. This is important in patient stratification and selection of therapy, especially the status of mediastinal and abdominal lymph nodes for the design of the field

for irradiation. It allows for maximizing dose delivery to areas of known disease.

REFERENCES

1. Edge SB, Byrd DR, Compton CC, et al, editors. AJCC cancer staging manual. 7th edition. New York: Springer; 2012. p. 129–49.
2. Rice TW, Rusch VW, Apperson-Hansen C, et al. Worldwide esophageal cancer collaboration (WECC). Dis Esophagus 2009;22:1–8.
3. NCCN clinical practice guidelines in oncology: esophageal and esophagogastric junction cancers version 2. 2011. Available at: www.nccn.org.
4. Krasna M, Ebright M. Overview. In: Sugarbaker DJ, editor. Adult chest surgery: concepts and procedures. New York: McGraw Hill; 2009. p. 98–9.
5. Krasna MJ. Esophageal cancer. BMJ 2012. Available at: https://online.epocrates.com/u/29111029/Esophageal+cancer.
6. Choi TK, Siu KF, Lam KH, et al. Bronchoscopy and carcinoma of the esophagus I. Findings of bronchoscopy in carcinoma of the esophagus. Am J Surg 1984;147:757–9.
7. Varghese T, Hofstetter W, Rizk N, et al. Guidelines on the diagnosis and staging of patients with esophageal cancer: workforce on evidence based surgery of the Society of Thoracic Surgeons. 2012. Available at: www.sts.org//EsophagealCancerDiagnosisStagingpdf/.
8. Esfandyari T, Potter JW, Vaezi MF. Dysphagia: a cost analysis of the diagnostic approach. Am J Gastroenterol 2002;97:2733–7.
9. van Vliet EP, Heijenbrok-Kal MH, Hunink MG, et al. Staging investigations for oesophageal cancer: a meta-analysis. Br J Cancer 2008;98(3):547–57.
10. Lefor AT, Merino MM, Steinberg SM, et al. Computerized tomographic prediction of extraluminal spread and prognostic implications of lesion width in esophageal carcinoma. Cancer 1988;62(7):1287–92.
11. Van Rossum PS, van Hillegersberg R, Lever FM, et al. Imaging strategies in the management of oesophageal cancer: what's the role of MRI? Eur Radiol 2013;23(7):1753–65.
12. Kato H, Nakajima M, Sohda M, et al. The clinical application of (18)F-fluorodeoxyglucose positron emission tomography to predict survival in patients with operable esophageal cancer. Cancer 2009; 115:3196–203.
13. Muijs CT, Beukema JC, Pruim J, et al. A systematic review on the role of FDG-PET/CT in tumour delineation and radiotherapy planning in patients with esophageal cancer. Radiother Oncol 2010;97(2): 165–71.
14. Wren SM, Stijns P, Srinivas S. Positron emission tomography in the initial staging of esophageal cancer. Arch Surg 2002;137:1001–6.

15. Yoon YC, Lee KS, Shim YM, et al. Metastasis to regional lymph nodes in patients with esophageal squamous cell carcinoma: CT versus FDG PET for presurgical detection – Prospective study. Radiology 2003;227:764–70.

16. Van Westreenen HL, Westerterp M, Bossuyt PM, et al. Systematic review of the staging performance of 18 F-fluorodeoxyglucose positron emission tomography in esophageal cancer. J Clin Oncol 2004;22(18):3805–12.

17. Walker AJ, Spier BJ, Perlman SB, et al. Integrated PET/CT fusion imaging and endoscopic ultrasound in the pre-operative staging and evaluation of esophageal cancer. Mol Imaging Biol 2011;13(1):166–71.

18. Choi J, Kim SG, Kim JS, et al. Comparison of endoscopic ultrasonography (EUS), positron emission tomography (PET) and computed tomography (CT) in the preoperative locoregional staging of resectable esophageal cancer. Surg Endosc 2010;24(6):1380–6.

19. Shan W, Kollmannsberger CK, Wilson D, et al. The utility of PET/CT in the treatment management of gastroesophageal cancer (GEC): impact on staging and treatment decisions. J Clin Oncol 2010;28(15). Suppl 1.

20. zum Büschenfelde CM, Herrmann K, Schuster T, et al. (18)F-FDG PET-guided salvage neoadjuvantradiochemotherapy of adenocarcinoma of the esophagogastric junction: the MUNICON II trial. J Nucl Med 2011;52:1189–96. http://dx.doi.org/10.2967/jnumed.110.085803.

21. Klaeser B, Nitzsche E, Schuller JC, et al. Limited predictive value of FDG-PET for response assessment in the preoperative treatment of esophageal cancer: results of a prospective multi-center trial (SAKK 75/02). Onkologie 2009;32:724–30.

22. Cerfolio RJ, Bryant AS, Ohja B, et al. The accuracy of endoscopic ultrasonography with fine-needle aspiration, integrated positron emission tomography with computed tomography, and computed tomography in restaging patients with esophageal cancer after neoadjuvantchemoradiotherapy. J Thorac Cardiovasc Surg 2005;129:1232–41.

23. Swisher SG, Erasmus J, Maish M, et al. 2-Fluoro-2-deoxy-D-glucose positron emission tomography imaging is predictive of pathologic response and survival after preoperative chemoradiation in patients with esophageal carcinoma. Cancer 2004;101:1776–85.

24. Ott K, Herrmann K, Krause BJ, et al. The value of PET imaging in patients with localized gastroesophageal cancer. Gastrointest Cancer Res 2008;2:287–94.

25. Puli SR, Reddy JB, Bechtold ML, et al. Staging accuracy of esophageal cancer by endoscopic ultrasound: a meta-analysis and systematic review. World J Gastroenterol 2008;14(10):1479–90.

26. Kelly S, Harri KM, Berry E, et al. A systematic review of the staging performance of endoscopic ultrasound in gastro-esophagal carcinoma. Gut 2001;49:534–9.

27. Lightdale CJ, Kulkarni KG. Role of endoscopic ultrasonograpy in the staging and follow-up of esophageal cancer. J Clin Oncol 2005;23:4483–9.

28. Sakano A, Yanai H, Sakaguchi E, et al. Clinical impact of tumor invasion depth staging of esophageal squamous cell carcinoma using endoscopic ultrasonography. Hepatogastroenterology 2010;57(104):1423–9.

29. Crabtree TD, Yacoub WN, Puri V, et al. Endoscopic ultrasound for early stage esophageal adenocarcinoma: implications for staging and survival. Ann Thorac Surg 2011;91:1509–16.

30. Eloubeidi MA, Cerfolio RJ, Bryant AS, et al. Efficacy of endoscopic ultrasound in patients with esophageal cancer predicted to have N0 disease. Eur J Cardiothorac Surg 2011;40(3):636–41.

31. Isenberg G, Chak A, Canto MI, et al. Endoscopic ultrasound in restaging of esophageal cancer after neoadjuvantchemoradiation. Gastrointest Endosc 1998;48:158–63.

32. Heinrich H, Bauerfeind P. Endoscopic mucosal resection for staging and therapy of adenocarcinoma of the esophagus, gastric cardia, and upper gastric third. Recent Results Cancer Res 2010;182:85–91.

33. Dagnini G, Caldironi MW, Marin G, et al. Laparoscopy in abdominal staging of esophageal carcinoma. Report of 369 cases. Gastrointest Endosc 1986;32(6):400–2.

34. Krasna MJ, Reed CE, Nedziecki D, et al. CALGB 9380: a prospective trial of feasibility of thoracoscopy/laparoscopy in staging esophageal cancer. Ann Thorac Surg 2001;71:1073–9.

35. Krasna MJ, Jiao X, Mao YS, et al. Thoracoscopy/laparoscopy in the staging of esophageal cancer. Surg Laparosc Endosc Percutan Tech 2002;12:213–8.

36. Romijn MG, van Overhagen H, Spillenaar Bilgen EJ, et al. Laparoscopy and laparoscopic ultrasonography in the staging of oesophageal and cardinal carcinoma. Br J Surg 1998;85:1010–2.

37. Bonavina L, Incarvone R, Lattuada E, et al. Preoperative laparoscopy in management of patients with carcinoma of the esophagus and of the esophagogastric junction. J Surg Oncol 1997;65:171–4.

38. Mezhir JJ, Shah MA, Jacks LM, et al. Positive peritoneal cytology in patients with gastric cancer: natural history and outcome of 291 patients. Ann Surg Oncol 2010;17(12):3173–80.

Esophageal Cancer Staging
Past, Present, and Future

Thomas W. Rice, MD[a],*, Eugene H. Blackstone, MD[b]

KEYWORDS

- T classification • N classification • M classification • Stage grouping • Histopathologic cell type
- Histologic grade • Cancer location • 7th edition AJCC Cancer Staging Manual

KEY POINTS

- TNM cancer staging describing anatomic extent of a cancer was developed between 1943 and 1952.
- TNM cancer staging was first applied to the esophagus in 1977.
- 7th edition esophageal cancer staging was data-driven, incorporated nonanatomic cancer characteristics, and harmonized with stomach cancer.
- 7th edition improvements include new definitions of Tis, T4, regional lymph node, N classification, and M classification, and the addition of nonanatomic cancer characteristics: histopathologic cell type, histologic grade, and cancer location.
- 8th edition esophageal cancer staging will address 6 problems in the continuing effort to improve and advance esophageal cancer staging.

THE PAST: TNM

The concept of TNM cancer staging describing the anatomic extent of a cancer was developed by Pierre Denoix at the Cancer Institute Gustave-Roussy between 1943 and 1952. It is based on the principle that as size of an untreated primary cancer (T) increases, regional lymph node metastases (N) and distant metastases (M) become more prevalent. Although introduced in 1953, it was not until 1968 that the first cancer staging manual was published by the International Union Against Cancer (UICC). In 1987, UICC and American Joint Committee on Cancer (AJCC) TNM classifications and stage groupings were unified. During the 42-year period from 1968 until publication of the 7th edition of the Cancer Staging Manual in 2010, revisions have been published every 6 to 8 years.

These revisions have been based on new knowledge, including improved understanding of cancer biology and factors affecting survival, and acquisition of clinical cancer data and new analytic techniques.

TNM esophageal cancer staging has had one of the slowest evolutions. It was first introduced by the UICC in 1968. In 1977, the 1st edition of the AJCC Manual for Staging Cancer introduced its TNM classifications (**Fig. 1**) and stage groupings (**Fig. 2**) for esophageal cancer.[1] For T1 and T2 cancers, T classification crudely expressed tumor area considering both cancer length and circumferential involvement. Only T3 cancers were grossly defined by depth of invasion, expressed only as extra-esophageal spread. Regional lymph node classification for thoracic esophageal cancers was a simple absent (N0) or present (N1)

The authors have nothing to disclose.
a Cleveland Clinic Lerner College of Medicine of Case Western Reserve University, and Heart and Vascular Institute, Department of Thoracic and Cardiovascular Surgery, 9500 Euclid Avenue, Desk J4-1, Cleveland, OH 44195, USA; b Cleveland Clinic Lerner College of Medicine of Case Western Reserve University, and Heart and Vascular Institute, Department of Thoracic and Cardiovascular Surgery, 9500 Euclid Avenue, Desk JJ-4, Cleveland, OH 44195, USA
* Corresponding author.
E-mail address: ricet@ccf.org

Thorac Surg Clin 23 (2013) 461–469
http://dx.doi.org/10.1016/j.thorsurg.2013.07.004
1547-4127/13/$ – see front matter © 2013 Elsevier Inc. All rights reserved.

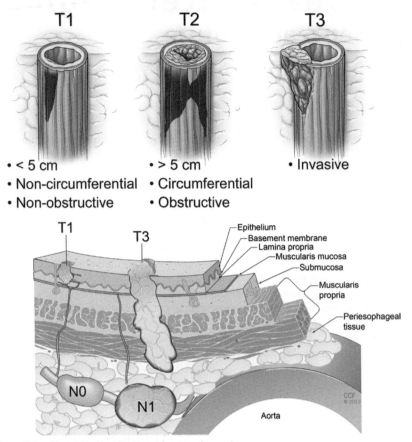

Fig. 1. 1997, 1st edition T and N classifications for esophageal cancer.

and remained so for 33 years through 6 editions. Distant metastases were either absent (M0) or present (M1). Clinical assessment of regional, cervical lymph nodes for cervical carcinoma was introduced, but eliminated by the 3rd edition.

The 2nd edition of AJCC TNM classifications was published in 1983; TNM classifications were unaltered, but stage groupings were extensively changed. The restriction of stage 0 to carcinoma

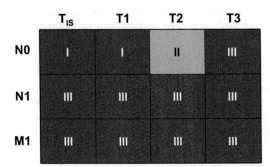

Fig. 2. 1997, 1st edition stage groupings for esophageal cancer.

in situ and stage IV to distant metastases was introduced.[2] These rigid definitions of stage 0 and IV, which remain today, were a regressive step because they limited options for stage groupings. A floor and ceiling were set, forcing all other cancers to be staged as I, II, or III. By survival analysis, some cancers at the outer extremes of stage I and III may best be grouped as stage 0 and IV, respectively, but are restricted from these groupings. This restriction decreases homogeneity of stage I and III, violating the principle of homogeneity of survival within stage groups.

In 1988, the 3rd edition of the AJCC Cancer Staging Manual dramatically changed esophageal cancer staging by reclassifying T only by depth of invasion (**Fig. 3**).[3] All regional lymph nodes (N) were still classified by either presence or absence of metastasis, and stage groupings were simplified (**Fig. 4**). There were no changes in esophageal cancer staging in the 1992 4th edition.[4] In 1997, the 5th edition introduced the subclassification of M1 into M1a (cervical lymph node metastasis for cancers of the upper thoracic esophagus and celiac lymph node metastasis for cancers of the

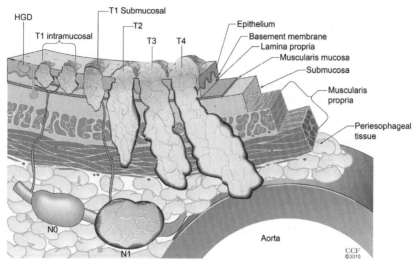

Fig. 3. 3rd through 6th edition T and N classifications for esophageal cancer.

lower thoracic esophagus) and M1b (all other distant metastases), and the subclassification of stage IV into IVA and IVB.[5] The 6th edition, published in 2002, was unchanged from the 5th edition.[6]

These prior editions of AJCC esophageal cancer staging were based on an empiric, simple, orderly arrangement of increasing pathologic anatomic T, then N, then M classifications, reflecting Denoix's basic principle. These stage groupings were not data-driven and did not take into account the growing body of literature concerning factors associated with survival, including both anatomic and nonanatomic cancer characteristics. Among these are the interplay of T and N and the prognostic importance of number of regional lymph nodes positive for cancer, histopathologic cell type, and histologic grade. In addition, the previous systems did not address cancers about the esophagogastric junction, nor differences in epidemiology and cancer characteristics between East and West.

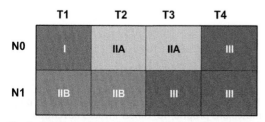

Fig. 4. 3rd through 6th edition stage groupings. Stage 0 (TisN0M0) and stage IV (Tany Nany M1), added in the 2nd edition stage groupings, are not shown. Similarly, stage IVA (Tany Nany M1a) and stage IVB (Tany Nany M1b), added in the 5th edition, are not shown.

THE PRESENT: 7TH EDITION

Although these prior staging manuals had been useful in treatment planning and prognostication, they were neither consistent with data nor biologically plausible. A radical change in esophageal cancer staging was necessary. Therefore, for the 7th edition, a data-driven, modern machine-learning analysis of a worldwide cancer experience was formulated.

Worldwide Esophageal Cancer Collaboration

At the request of the AJCC, the Worldwide Esophageal Cancer Collaboration (WECC) was inaugurated in 2006. Thirteen institutions from 5 countries and 3 continents (Asia, Europe, and North America) submitted de-identified data by July 2007. These de-identified data were used to construct a database of 4627 esophagectomy patients who had no induction or adjuvant therapy.[7]

Modern Machine-Learning Analysis

Multiple previously proposed revisions of esophageal cancer staging have examined goodness of fit or P values to test for a statistically significant effect of stage on survival. Instead, staging for the 7th edition used random forest (RF) analysis, a machine-learning technique that focuses on predictiveness for future patients.[8] RF analysis makes no a priori assumptions about patient survival, is able to identify complex interactions among variables, and accounts for nonlinear effects.

RF analysis first isolated cancer characteristics of interest from other factors influencing survival by generating risk-adjusted survival curves for each patient. Unlike previous approaches that began by placing cancer characteristics into proposed groups, RF analysis produced distinct groups with monotonically decreasing risk-adjusted survival without regard to cancer characteristics. Then, anatomic and nonanatomic cancer characteristics important for stage group composition were identified within these groups. Finally, homogeneity within groups guided both amalgamation and segmentation of cancer characteristics between adjacent groups to arrive at the final stage groups. This data-driven effort produced the 7th edition cancer staging recommendations.[9–12]

7th Edition: TNM Classification Changes and Additions

This 7th edition analysis resulted in the following classifications (**Fig. 5** and **Box 1**).[9–12] T classification is changed for Tis and T4 cancers. Tis is now defined as high-grade dysplasia and includes all noninvasive neoplastic epithelium that was previously called carcinoma in situ. T4, tumors invading local structures, are subclassified as T4a and T4b. T4a tumors are resectable cancers invading adjacent structures, such as the pleura, pericardium, or diaphragm; T4b tumors are unresectable cancers invading other adjacent structures, such as

the aorta, vertebral body, and trachea. T1 through T3 subclassifications are unchanged.

A regional lymph node is redefined to include any paraesophageal node extending from cervical nodes to celiac nodes. In classifying N, the data support convenient coarse groupings of number of cancer-positive nodes (0, 1–2, 3–6, 7 or more). These groupings are designated N0 (none), N1 (1–2), N2 (3–6), and N3 (7 or more) and are identical to gastric N classifications (see **Fig. 5** and **Box 1**).

The subclassifications M1a and M1b are eliminated, as is MX (see **Fig. 5** and **Box 1**). Distant metastasis is simply designated M0, no distant metastasis, and M1, distant metastasis.

7th Edition: Nonanatomic Cancer Characteristics

Nonanatomic classifications identified as important for stage grouping are histopathologic cell type (see **Box 1**), histologic grade (see **Box 1**), and tumor location (see **Fig. 6** and **Box 1**). The difference in survival between adenocarcinoma and squamous cell carcinoma is best managed by separate stage groupings for stages I and II. Increasing histologic grade is associated with incrementally decreasing survival for early-stage cancers. For adenocarcinoma, distinguishing G1 and G2 (well and moderately differentiated) from

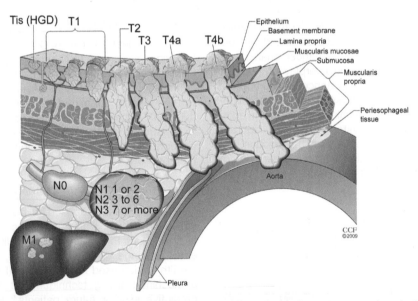

Fig. 5. 7th edition TNM classifications. T is classified as Tis, high-grade dysplasia; T1, cancer invades lamina propria, muscularis mucosae, or submucosa; T2, cancer invades muscularis propria; T3, cancer invades adventitia; T4a, resectable cancer invades adjacent structures, such as pleura, pericardium, or diaphragm; T4b, unresectable cancer invades other adjacent structures, such as aorta, vertebral body, or trachea. N is classified as N0, no regional lymph node metastasis; N1, regional lymph node metastases involving 1 to 2 nodes; N2, regional lymph node metastases involving 3 to 6 nodes; N3, regional lymph node metastases involving 7 or more nodes. M is classified as M0, no distant metastasis; M1, distant metastasis.

Box 1
Summary of changes in anatomic classifications and additions of nonanatomic cancer characteristics in the 7th edition

Changes in anatomic classifications

T classification

Tis is redefined and T4 is subclassified

Tis: high-grade dysplasia

T4a: resectable cancer invades adjacent structures, such as pleura, pericardium, diaphragm

T4b: unresectable cancer invades adjacent structures, such as aorta, vertebral body, trachea

N classification

Regional lymph node is redefined

Any periesophageal lymph node from cervical lymph nodes to celiac node

N is classified

N0: no regional lymph node metastases

N1: 1 to 2 positive regional lymph nodes

N2: 3 to 6 positive regional lymph nodes

N3: 7 or more positive regional lymph nodes

M classification

M is redefined

M0: no distant metastases

M1: distant metastases

Additions of nonanatomic cancer characteristics

Histopathologic cell type

Adenocarcinoma

Squamous cell carcinoma

Histologic grade

G1: well differentiated

G2: moderately differentiated

G3: poorly differentiated

G4: undifferentiated

Cancer location

Upper thoracic: 20 to 25 cm from incisors

Middle thoracic: >25 to 30 cm from incisors

Lower thoracic: >30 to 40 cm from incisors

Esophagogastric junction includes cancers whose epicenter is (1) in the lower thoracic esophagus, (2) in the esophagogastric junction, or (3) within proximal 5 cm of the stomach (cardia) that extend into the esophagogastric junction or lower thoracic esophagus

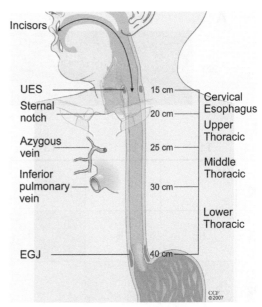

Fig. 6. Cancer location. Cervical esophagus, bounded superiorly by the cricopharyngeus and inferiorly by the sternal notch, is typically 15 to 20 cm from the incisors at esophagoscopy. Upper thoracic esophagus, bounded superiorly by the sternal notch and inferiorly by the azygos arch, is typically greater than 20 to 25 cm from the incisors at esophagoscopy. Middle thoracic esophagus, bounded superiorly by the azygos arch and inferiorly by the inferior pulmonary vein, is typically greater than 25 to 30 cm from the incisors at esophagoscopy. Lower thoracic esophagus, bounded superiorly by the inferior pulmonary vein and inferiorly by the lower esophageal sphincter, is typically greater than 30 to 40 cm from the incisors at esophagoscopy; it includes cancers whose epicenter is within the proximal 5 cm of the stomach that extend into the esophagogastric junction or lower thoracic esophagus.

G3 (poorly differentiated) is important for stage I and stage IIA cancers. For squamous cell carcinoma, distinguishing G1 from G2 and G3 is important for stage I and II cancers. Tumor location (upper and middle thoracic vs lower thoracic) is important for grouping T2-3N0M0 squamous cell cancers.

7th Edition: Stage Groupings

Stages 0 and IV are by definition (not data-driven) TisN0M0 and T, any N, any M1, respectively. For T1N0M0 and T2N0M0 adenocarcinoma, subgrouping is by histologic grade: not G3 (G1 and G2) versus G3 (**Fig. 7**A). Stage groupings for the remainder of M0 adenocarcinomas are shown in **Fig. 7**B.

For T1N0M0 squamous cell carcinoma, subgrouping is by histologic grade: G1 versus not

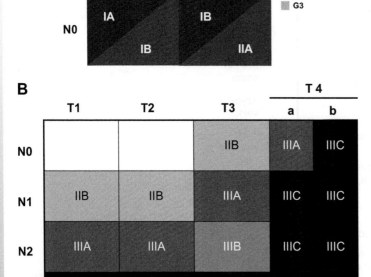

Fig. 7. Stage groupings for M0 adenocarcinoma. (*A*) Stage groupings for T1N0M0 and T2N0M0 by T and N classification and histologic grade (G). (*B*) Stage groupings for other M0 adenocarcinomas.

G1 (G2 and G3) (**Fig. 8**A). For T2N0M0 and T3N0M0 squamous cell carcinoma, stage grouping is by histologic grade and location (see **Fig. 8**B). The 4 combinations range from G1 lower thoracic squamous cell carcinoma (stage IB), which has the best survival, to G2-G3 upper and middle thoracic squamous cell carcinomas (stage IIB), which have the worst. G2-G3 lower thoracic squamous cell carcinomas and G1 upper and middle thoracic squamous cell carcinomas are grouped together (stage IIA), with intermediate survival. Stage groupings for the remainder of M0 squamous cell carcinomas are shown in **Fig. 8**C.

Stage 0, III, and IV adenocarcinoma and squamous cell carcinoma are identically stage grouped. Adenosquamous carcinomas are staged as squamous cell carcinoma.

7th Edition: Esophagogastric Junction Cancers

Besides being data-driven, the 2010 7th edition staging system harmonizes staging of cancer across the esophagogastric junction. Previous staging produced different stage groupings for these cancers, depending on the use of either esophageal or gastric stage groupings. The 2010 AJCC/UICC staging is for cancers of the esophagus and esophagogastric junction and includes cancer within the first 5 cm of the stomach (cardia) that invade the esophagogastric junction (Siewert III).

The Future: 8th Edition and Beyond

The 7th edition heralded the era of data-driven cancer staging and will serve as the foundation for future staging.[13] However, this edition was based on only esophagectomy data, an obvious shortcoming. Improvements in the next iterations of esophageal cancer staging will require the following:

1. Obtaining better homogeneity of stage 0 and stage IV. This will require abandoning restrictive definitions of these stage groupings and changing composition of adjacent stage IA and stage IIIC (**Figs. 9** and **10**).
2. Improving homogeneity of stage IIB adenocarcinoma (see **Fig. 9**) and stage IIA and IIB squamous cell cancer (see **Fig. 10**). This will require expanding the WECC database of these less common cancers.
3. Adding clinical (cStage), postinduction clinical and postdefinitive nonsurgical clinical (ycStage), and post-induction pathologic (ypStage) staging recommendations. This will require expanding the data analysis.

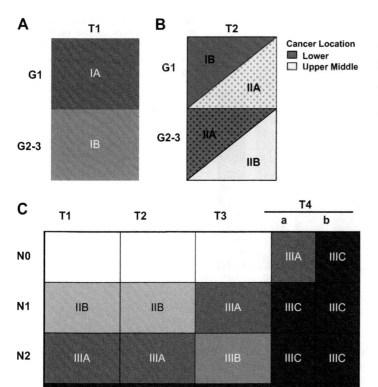

Fig. 8. Stage groupings for M0 squamous cell carcinoma. (*A*) Stage groupings for T1N0M0 by histologic grade (G). (*B*) Stage groupings for T2-3N0M0 by histologic grade (G) and cancer location. (*C*) Stage groupings for other M0 squamous cell carcinomas.

4. Assessing other nonanatomic tumor characteristics that affect survival. This will require expanding data elements beyond histopathologic cell type, histologic grade, and cancer location.

5. Adding nonesophagectomy survival data, endoscopic treatment in stage 0 and stage IA, and palliative therapy for stage IV, which will require partnering with nonsurgical specialties and professional associations and groups.

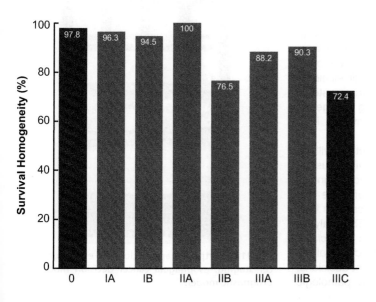

Fig. 9. 7th edition staging of adenocarcinoma of the esophagus: a measure of homogeneity within stage groupings with respect to survival.

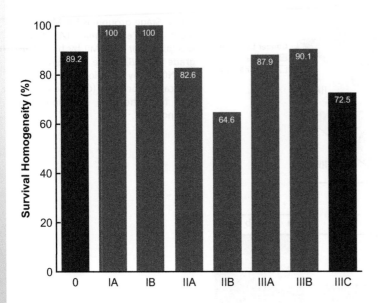

Fig. 10. 7th edition staging of squamous cell cancer of the esophagus: a measure of homogeneity within stage groupings with respect to survival.

6. Adding cancer of the cervical esophagus. This will require partnering and harmonizing with the head and neck task force, mirroring the process used with the gastric cancer task force for the 7th edition.

Acquisition of multicenter, international data through WECC is key to this effort.[7] Innovative machine learning techniques will again be used for analysis.[8] The strategy for adding clinical, postinduction, and definitive nonoperative therapy and postinduction pathologic staging will be to reference these stages to the 8th edition pStaging platform.

BEYOND ANATOMIC STAGING

Differences in the focus and goals of the AJCC and UICC in cancer staging may be obviated by extinction of the printed manual and development of an Internet cancer staging site. This will eliminate the need for a blanket change to all organ systems every 6 to 7 years, permitting ongoing changes to each organ system when adjustments are indicated and necessary.

Use of patient and treatment factors will be expanded in future analyses that will focus on the individual patient. Patient-specific prognosis requires more than risk adjustment of these factors (used in the 7th edition); it necessitates their addition as variables in the analyses. The analyses will provide the 2 following models: a *decision model* based on clinical staging and additional patient factors that will assist in treatment decisions, and a *prognostic model* based on pathologic

staging, patient factors, and treatment delivered that will facilitate prognostication. Smartphone applications or their equivalent are envisioned for patient and physician use (**Fig. 11**).

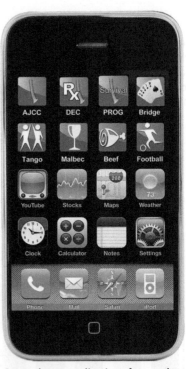

Fig. 11. Smartphone applications for esophageal cancer staging: esophageal cancer decision model and prognostic model.

SUMMARY

The concept of TNM cancer staging describing the anatomic extent of a cancer was developed between 1943 and 1952. However, it was not applied to esophageal cancer until 1977. The faithful adherences to the empiric staging process that was based on the stepwise progression of increasing local cancer invasion (T), followed by metastases to regional lymph nodes (N), and finally metastases to distant sites (M) dominated esophageal cancer staging for the next 33 years, through 6 editions.

The 7th edition staging recommendations for cancer of the esophagus and esophagogastric junction are data-driven and harmonized with stomach cancer, which required changes in TNM definitions and addition of nonanatomic cancer characteristics. For cancers of the esophagus and esophagogastric junction, stages 0, III, and IV are identical for both adenocarcinoma and squamous cell carcinoma. However, stage groupings differ for stage I and II cancers based on histopathologic cell type, histologic grade, and cancer location.

Improving cancer staging requires a release from the strict TNM description of anatomic staging. The inclusion of TNM variables with others (to be identified) will allow a more complete definition of the esophageal cancer, and aid in treatment decisions, and facilitate prognostication.

REFERENCES

1. Staging of cancer of the esophagus. In: Beahrs OH, Carr DT, Rubin P, editors. Manual for staging of cancer. 1st edition. Philadelphia: JB Lippincott; 1977. p. 65–70.
2. Esophagus. In: Beahrs OH, Myers MH, editors. Manual for staging of cancer. 2nd edition. Philadelphia: JB Lippincott; 1983. p. 61–6.
3. Esophagus. In: Beahrs OH, Henson DE, Hutter RV, et al, editors. Manual for staging of cancer. 3rd edition. Philadelphia: JB Lippincott; 1988. p. 63–7.
4. Esophagus. In: Beahrs OH, Henson DE, Hutter RV, et al, editors. Manual for staging of cancer. 4th edition. Philadelphia: JB Lippincott; 1992. p. 63–7.
5. Esophagus. In: Fleming ID, Cooper JS, Henson DE, et al, editors. AJCC cancer staging manual. 5th edition. Philadelphia: Lippincott-Raven; 1997. p. 65–9.
6. Esophagus. In: Greene FL, Page DL, Fleming ID, et al, editors. AJCC cancer staging manual. 6th edition. New York: Springer; 2002. p. 91–8.
7. Rice TW, Rusch VW, Apperson-Hansen C, et al. Worldwide esophageal cancer collaboration. Dis Esophagus 2009;22:1–8.
8. Ishwaran H, Blackstone EH, Apperson-Hansen C, et al. A novel approach to cancer staging: application to esophageal cancer. Biostatistics 2009;10:603–20.
9. Rice TW, Rusch VW, Ishwaran H, et al. Cancer of the esophagus and esophagogastric junction: data-driven staging for the 7th edition of the AJCC cancer staging manual. Cancer 2010;16:3763–73.
10. Esophagus and esophagogastric junction. In: Edge SB, Byrd DR, Compton CC, et al, editors. AJCC cancer staging manual. 7th edition. New York: Springer; 2010. p. 103–15.
11. Oesophagus including oesophagogastric junction. International Union Against Cancer: TNM classification of malignant tumours. 7th edition. Oxford (United Kingdom): Wiley-Blackwell; 2009. p. 66–72.
12. Rice TW, Blackstone EH, Rusch VW. A cancer staging primer: esophagus and esophagogastric junction. J Thorac Cardiovasc Surg 2010;139:527–9.
13. Rusch VW, Rice TW, Crowley J, et al. The seventh edition of the American Joint Committee on Cancer/International Union Against Cancer Staging Manuals: the new era of data-driven revisions. J Thorac Cardiovasc Surg 2010;139:819–21.

Personalizing Therapy for Esophageal Cancer Patients

Toshitaka Hoppo, MD, PhD, Blair A. Jobe, MD*

KEYWORDS

- Esophageal cancer • Endoscopy • Esophagectomy • Diagnosis • Therapy

KEY POINTS

- The management of esophageal cancer starts with accurate tissue diagnosis and clinical staging.
- Advances in screening and surveillance programs and endoscopic techniques have resulted in patients with early-stage esophageal cancer diagnosed more frequently.
- *Endoscopic mucosal resection* (EMR) for staging purposes is essential to diagnose T1a cancer and crucial to exclude risk factors for progression to cancer or presence of concomitant cancer.
- Esophagectomy plays a major role as an essential component of treatment in patients with locally advanced, resectable esophageal cancer.
- Despite intensive multidisciplinary approaches, including surgery, chemotherapy, and radiotherapy, the prognosis of esophageal cancer is unacceptable.
- There remains room for improvements in treatment strategies and optimal regimens of neoadjuvant and adjuvant therapy.

INTRODUCTION

Over the past several decades, the incidence of esophageal cancer, especially esophageal adenocarcinoma, has been dramatically increasing in Western countries, and the prognosis remains unacceptable, with a 5-year survival rate of approximately 15% despite multidisciplinary approaches, including neoadjuvant and adjuvant chemoradiation and surgical therapy.[1,2] Barrett esophagus (BE) has been recognized as a risk factor for esophageal adenocarcinoma, and esophageal carcinogenesis from metaplasia through dysplasia to adenocarcinoma has been extensively investigated and accepted.[3,4] High-grade dysplasia (HGD) has the highest risk of progression to adenocarcinoma, although the natural history of HGD remains unclear. Based on previous studies demonstrating that concomitant cancer was found in approximately 40% of surgically resected specimens of

patients who had a preoperative diagnosis of only HGD,[5,6] surgical resection of the esophagus (esophagectomy) has been recommended as standard of care. Esophagectomy is one of the most complex procedures used in the gastrointestinal tract, and its mortality rate may exceed 3%.[7,8] Several studies have demonstrated the majority of patients who present with HGD and are subsequently discovered to have synchronous cancer do not have invasion into the submucosa (ie, T1a). The probability of lymph node involvement in patients with intramucosal adenocarcinoma is unlikely (<2%), suggesting that esophagectomy in this setting may be unreasonably invasive.[9–11]

With recent advances in endoscopic imaging and surveillance and endoscopic therapeutic techniques, patients with HGD and/or early esophageal cancer have been increasingly recognized.[12,13] Selected patients with HGD and/or early cancer have been successfully treated with

Disclosures: The authors have nothing to disclose.
Department of Surgery, Institute for the Treatment of Esophageal and Thoracic Disease, The Western Pennsylvania Hospital, Allegheny Health Network, 4600 Friendship Avenue, Suite 4800, Pittsburgh, PA 15224, USA
* Corresponding author.
E-mail address: bjobe1@wpahs.org

Thorac Surg Clin 23 (2013) 471–478
http://dx.doi.org/10.1016/j.thorsurg.2013.07.001
1547-4127/13/$ – see front matter © 2013 Elsevier Inc. All rights reserved

esophageal-preserving endoscopic therapy, including endoscopic ablation (radiofrequency ablation and cryotherapy) and resection (EMR and endoscopic submucosal dissection), with oncological outcomes equivalent to those of surgical resection.[14,15] Esophageal-preserving therapy indicates any endoluminal procedure that is performed in an attempt to completely eradicate disease while preserving the anatomic structure of esophagus. The guidelines put forth by the American College of Gastroenterology (2008) state that esophagectomy is no longer the necessary treatment response to HGD[16]; however, the optimal management of HGD and/or early esophageal cancer remains controversial. Accumulating data have suggested that esophageal-preserving therapy can be a reasonable option in highly selected patients with HGD and/or early esophageal cancer with low risk or no risk of lymph node involvement, causing more confusion in the decision making of health care providers. In contrast, there is no doubt that esophagectomy plays a major role as an essential component of treatment in patients with locally advanced, resectable esophageal cancer without evidence of metastatic disease. This article focuses on the process of decision making used to select the optimal therapy for a given patient with esophageal cancer.

PATIENT SELECTION AND CLINICAL STAGING

The management of esophageal cancer starts with meticulous, endoscopic examination of esophageal epithelium with extensive biopsies for tissue diagnosis and staging EMR to determine the depth of tumor invasion if there is a nodule present. The Seattle protocol (biopsies with jumbo forceps in 4 quadrants, along every centimeter of endoscopically apparent disease with additional biopsies taken from suspicious areas) has been widely used[17]; however, only 2% of the total surface area of esophageal epithelium at a given level is obtained for histologic examination using this protocol and most areas are not histologically examined, causing the potential for sampling error, especially in patients with long-segment BE. Therefore, having high-quality endoscopic images is important to detect questionable, subtle mucosal abnormalities. Several new endoscopic technologies (eg, confocal laser endomicroscopy, autofluorescent imaging, and optical coherent tomography) combined with enhancement techniques (eg, narrow band imaging and chromoendoscopy) have been investigated for more efficient endoscopic examination; however, none of these technologies has been routinely used

in general practice by the gastroenterology community at large. Histologic determination of dysplasia (in particular, low-grade dysplasia) is significantly associated with interobserver variability among pathologists, and review by 2 experienced pathologists are recommended to confirm histology of dysplasia.[18,19]

To complete clinical staging, all patients with esophageal cancer require positron emission tomography/CT for the assessment of metastatic disease and endoscopic ultrasound (EUS) for the assessment of tumor depth and lymph node involvement. A meta-analysis has demonstrated that the pooled sensitivity and specificity of EUS to diagnose T1 stage cancer was 81.6% and 99.4%, respectively,[20] suggesting that EUS cannot discriminate accurately between T1a and T1b esophageal cancers, even with high-frequency miniprobe (20–30 MHz).[21] For the accurate diagnosis of T1a cancer, staging EMR is essential, and it is particularly important to exclude submucosal invasion (T1b) and any possibility of lymph node involvement and metastatic disease when esophageal-preserving therapy is considered. Esophageal-preserving therapy should be indicated only for patients with HGD and/or T1a cancer at present or those with T1b lesions and poor functional status. For locally advanced resectable cancers, esophagectomy with or without neoadjuvant and/or adjuvant chemoradiation therapy (CRT) has been the most common approach, although the optimal neoadjuvant/adjuvant treatment regimen has not been established. For unresectable cancers, nonsurgical treatment with CRT can be an option; however, palliative care may be more important than any curative treatments, with a particular emphasis on the alleviation of dysphagia using endoscopic techniques and radiation (to remedy chronic blood loss from the primary tumor). The algorithm of decision making is summarized in **Fig. 1**.

HGD AND T1A ESOPHAGEAL CANCER

A previous prospective study has demonstrated that patients with HGD and/or T1a esophageal cancer (n = 349) have a low risk of lymph node involvement and can be safely and successfully treated with esophageal-preserving therapy, including endoscopic ablation and resection, with excellent long-term (5 years) and complete remission rates of more than 95% without tumor-related deaths.[14] Furthermore, patients who completed eradication of esophageal neoplasia and subsequently received radiofrequency ablation therapy for persistent or recurrent BE had a lower incidence of metachronous neoplasia

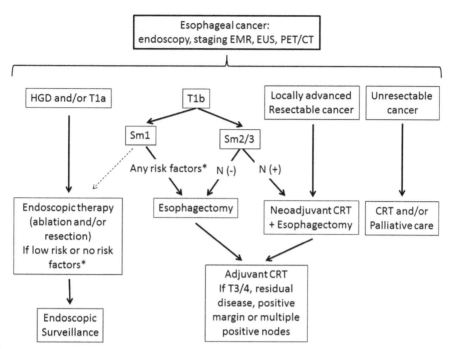

Fig. 1. Algorithm of decision making based on clinical staging. *Risk factors are summarized in **Table 1**.

during follow-up compared with those who did not receive ablation therapy (16.5% vs 29.9%).[14] These data suggest that additional ablative therapy for remaining BE may reduce the development of metachronous neoplasia. Piecemeal resection, long-segment BE, no ablation therapy of remaining nondysplastic BE, multifocal neoplasia, and a long time (>10 months) to achieve an initial complete response are independent risk factors associated recurrence after a complete local response.[14] The recent systematic review involving 1874 patients who had esophagectomy for the treatment of HGD and/or T1a cancer demonstrates that no metastatic disease was found in patients with HGD and 1.93% of patients with T1a cancer had positive lymph nodes, which was lower than the rate of mortality and morbidity observed with esophagectomy.[22] When esophageal-preserving therapy is considered, it is critical to exclude patients at high risk for progression to cancer or presence of concomitant cancer with potential lymph node involvement. Previous studies have demonstrated that patients with multifocal HGD have a high risk of concomitant cancer, ranging from 60% to 78%, whereas limited or focal HGD is less likely associated with concomitant cancer or progression to cancer.[12,13,23,24] This suggests that patients with multifocal HGD require meticulous endoscopic examination with extensive biopsies (and endoscopic resection of nodules) to reduce the

probability of sampling error and establish accurate clinical staging (ie, T1a vs T1b) before esophageal-preserving therapy is considered. Submucosal invasion (T1b), squamous-type histology, lymphovascular invasion (L+ or V+), poor differentiation, and a nodule greater than 3 cm in diameter are all associated with an increased risk of lymph node involvement (**Table 1**).[25–28]

Successful esophageal-preserving therapy is highly dependent on intensive follow-up and strict acid suppression with high-dose proton pump inhibitor and nocturnal H_2-blocker, which establish an acid-free environment in the treated area, thus facilitating the healing process to the normal neosquamous lining. There is no consensus on optimal protocol for surveillance after esophageal-preserving therapy; however, the guidelines issued by the American Society for Gastrointestinal Endoscopy (ASGE) state that patients with HGD should undergo surveillance endoscopy every 3 months for at least 1 year, with multiple large-capacity biopsy specimens obtained at 1-cm intervals. After 1 year, if there is no detection of recurrence, the interval of surveillance may be lengthened if there are no dysplastic changes on 2 subsequent endoscopies performed at 3-month intervals.[29] BE results from long-term acid exposure to the distal esophagus and a surgical repair to prevent gastroesophageal reflux could, therefore, minimize the development

Table 1
Risk factors to consider for esophageal-preserving therapy

Low Risk	High Risk
Concurrent cancer or progression to invasive cancer	
Unifocal (limited or focal), flat HGD	Multifocal HGD, HGD with nodules
Lymph node involvement	
Type I, type IIa <20 mm, type IIb, type IIc <10 mm	Type I, type II >30 mm, type III
Well or moderately differentiated adenocarcinoma (grading G1/G2)	Poorly differentiated adenocarcinoma (grading G3), squamous cell carcinoma
Lesions limited to the mucosa (m)	Invasion into submucosal layer (sm)
No lymphovascular invasion	Presence of lymphovasuclar invasion

Abbreviations: Type I, polypoid type; type II, flat type; type IIa, flat, elevated; type IIb, level with the mucosa; type IIc, slightly depressed; type III, ulcerated type.

Data from Hoppo T, Rachit SD, Jobe BA. Esophageal preservation in esophageal high-grade dysplasia and intramucosal adenocarcinoma. Thorac Surg Clin 2011; 21(4):528, with permission; and Japanese Gastric Cancer Association. Japanese classification of gastric carcinoma - 2nd English edition. Gastric Cancer 1998;1(1):10–24.

of cancer or recurrence of BE.[30] There have been, however, no adequately powered studies to support this hypothesis because of the low incidence of esophageal cancer. Although the ASGE guidelines state that antireflux surgery should not be advised, with the rationale that the procedure prevents esophageal cancer,[29] antireflux surgery is worth considering to eliminate all acid exposure and usage of antisecretory medications, once the eradication of HGD is confirmed. Based on the ASGE guideline, it may be reasonable to perform intensive surveillance every 3 months up to 1 year after esophageal-preserving therapy and then consider antireflux surgery if there is no evidence of recurrence. Long-term endoscopic surveillance, however, per ASGE guidelines, is still required regardless of whether antireflux surgery is used. If BE is refractory to endoscopic ablation and resection (particularly at the level of esophagogastric junction), the continuous acid exposure to the distal esophagus via significant gastroesophageal reflux may affect the healing process from endoscopic therapy. In

such cases, it is worth considering antireflux surgery to treat the underlying gastroesophageal reflux disease and then continuing endoscopic surveillance with additional ablation or resection.

T1B ESOPHAGEAL CANCER

Once tumors invade the submucosal layer, the possibility of lymph node involvement is exponentially increased due to the abundant submucosal lymphatic network,[31,32] and esophagectomy has, therefore, been recommended as a standard of care for T1b submucosal cancer. For more accurate staging purposes, the mucosal and submucosal layers have been subdivided into thirds with each third going deeper into the esophageal wall, and T1 cancers have 6 different layers of invasion: T1m1 to T1m3 (m1: limited to the epithelial layer, m2: invades lamina propria, m3: invades into but not through muscularis mucosae) and T1sm1 to T1sm3 (even thirds of the submucosa). In a recent review using the pooled data of 7645 patients with T1b submucosal esophageal cancer, Gockel and colleagues[33] reported that the overall rate of lymph node involvement in submucosal cancer was 37%; however, there was a substantial difference between T1sm1 and T1sm2/3 (6% vs 23%/58%, respectively), suggesting that highly selected T1sm1 adenocarcinoma lesions could be treated by esophageal-preserving therapy. This is further supported by the most recent study involving 66 patients with low-risk T1sm1 cancer (macroscopically polypoid or flat lesion, well-to-moderate differentiation, and no lymphovascular invasion), demonstrating that 97% of patients with small nodules less than or equal to 2 cm achieved complete remission and 90% of those achieved long-term remission without the development of metachronous disease. Although 1 patient developed lymph node metastasis, no tumor-associated deaths were observed and the estimated 5-year survival of this cohort was 84%.[34] The risk of developing lymph node metastasis after esophageal-preserving therapy for T1sm1 seems lower than the risk of esophagectomy, suggesting that patients with low-risk T1sm1 could also be reasonable candidates for esophageal-preserving therapy, particularly when poor functional status and comorbid conditions make esophageal resection too risky. In contrast, T1sm2 and T1sm3 are associated with the high rate of lymph node involvement, and esophagectomy should be considered.[35,36] There is likely a publication bias to these data, however, because results were achieved within high-volume centers of excellence. These results may not be transferrable to patients at all centers delivering therapy.

LOCALLY ADVANCED ESOPHAGEAL CANCER

For patients with locally advanced, resectable esophageal cancer, the most common approaches include neoadjuvant chemotherapy or chemoradiation, surgery, and adjuvant CRT. Provided they have adequate performance status, surgical resection is an essential component of the treatment plan in patients with locally advanced esophageal cancer without evidence of metastatic disease. The purpose of neoadjuvant therapy is to achieve tumor down-staging and thus increase the probability of R0 resection and minimize local recurrence. Several randomized controlled studies comparing neoadjuvant chemoradiation (CRT) therapy followed by surgery versus surgery alone have suggested better local control and 2-year and 5-year survival rates with neoadjuvant CRT followed by surgery.[37–40] Walsh and colleagues[40] have reported that a complete histologic response was achieved in approximately 25% of patients who had undergone neoadjuvant CRT therapy, and regional nodal involvement was less frequent in the CRT group (42% vs 82%). Neoadjuvant CRT was associated with significantly longer median survival (16 months vs 11 months) and 3-year survival (32% vs 6%). In another study involving 56 patients, Tepper and colleagues[38] reported that a complete histologic response was achieved in approximately 40% of patients who had undergone neoadjuvant CRT, and 5-year survival was significantly improved in the CRT group (39% vs 16%). This study, however, was underpowered. In the most recent phase III Dutch study (the CROSS study), patients in the CRT group underwent a new regimen of carboplatin and paclitaxel for 5 weeks and concurrent radiation therapy (41 Gy) followed by surgery, 29% of whom achieved a pathologic complete response. R0 resection was achieved in 92% of patients in the CRT group as opposed to 69% in the surgery alone group ($P<.001$) with similar postoperative mortality and morbidity rates. The CRT group had significantly better median overall survival compared with the surgery alone group (49.4 vs 24 months, $P = .003$).[41] Furthermore, the recent meta-analysis of pooled data involving 4188 patients who had undergone neoadjuvant therapy (chemotherapy and chemoradiation) demonstrated a survival benefit of neoadjuvant chemotherapy or CRT over surgery alone, although there was no significant difference between neoadjuvant chemotherapy versus CRT.[42] Based on these data, neoadjuvant therapy prior to surgery has been recommended for patients with greater than T1 disease or node-positive disease, although the optimal neoadjuvant regimen has not been established.

The purpose of adjuvant therapy is to minimize the risk of local and systemic recurrence and to attempt to improve survival, especially in patients with T3 or T4 tumors, residual disease, microscopically positive margin, or multiple positive nodes. Several phase III trials comparing adjuvant radiotherapy with surgery alone have demonstrated improved local control with adjuvant radiotherapy but no survival benefit.[43,44] A phase III study that compared adjuvant radiotherapy with adjuvant chemotherapy demonstrated no significant difference in 5-year survival or local recurrence rates.[45] In a randomized controlled trial comparing adjuvant CRT with surgery alone (the INT-0016 trial), MacDonald and colleagues[46] demonstrated a significantly improved 3-year survival (50% vs 41%) and median duration of relapse-free survival (30 vs 19 months) in the CRT group. In addition, the rate of local recurrence was lower in the CRT group (19% vs 29%). Based on these data, adjuvant CRT should be considered for patients with T3 or T4 tumors, residual disease, microscopically positive margin, or multiple positive nodes. The actual benefit of adjuvant therapy in patients who are nonresponders to neoadjuvant therapy remains unclear.

Recent advances in understanding the molecular biology of cancer have led to the development of targeted systemic therapies that work to disrupt specific mechanisms involved in carcinogenesis, such as cellular growth protein receptors and downstream signaling pathways. The advantage of targeted therapy is that it potentially minimizes medication-related side effects and improves efficacy. These agents include epidermal growth factor receptor (ErbB-1 and HER-2)[47,48] and vascular endothelial growth factor antagonists.[49] Further studies are required to evaluate the therapeutic efficacy of these approaches.

UNRESECTABLE ESOPHAGEAL CANCER

For patients with advanced unresectable esophageal cancer with or without metastatic disease, nonsurgical treatment with CRT has been recommended since the Radiation Therapy Oncology Group 85-01 trial comparing CRT with radiotherapy alone, which demonstrated that CRT increased the 5-year survival compared with radiotherapy alone (26% vs 0%).[50,51] In this situation, patients may have intractable symptoms, such as dysphagia, nausea, vomiting, pain, and dyspnea, significantly affecting their quality of life. Symptom management and improvement in quality of life may be more important than treatments aimed with curative intent, which may be no longer available or desired.

SUMMARY

The management of esophageal cancer starts with accurate tissue diagnosis and clinical staging. With advances in screening and surveillance programs and endoscopic techniques, patients with early-stage esophageal cancer have been diagnosed more frequently, and esophageal-preserving therapy can be used for those with a low-risk of lymph node involvement. EMR for staging purposes is essential to diagnose T1a cancer, and it is crucial to exclude risk factors for progression to cancer or presence of concomitant cancer. The treatment of T1b cancer remains controversial; however, superficial T1b (sm1) with low-risk factors (polypoid or flat lesion ≤2 cm, no lymphovascular invasion, well differentiated, or moderately differentiated) could be treated by esophageal-preserving therapy. Esophagectomy plays a major role as an essential component of treatment in patients with locally advanced, resectable esophageal cancer. Neoadjuvant and adjuvant CRT seem to improve survival and minimize local recurrence, although the optimal neoadjuvant and adjuvant regimen has not been established. Patients with unresectable cancer may benefit from CRT; however, palliative care may be more important for symptom management and improvement in quality of life. Despite intensive multidisciplinary approaches including surgery, chemotherapy, and radiotherapy, the prognosis of esophageal cancer is unacceptable. There remains room for improvements in treatment strategies and optimal regimens of neoadjuvant and adjuvant therapy. In this context, it is particularly important to find early-stage disease and initiate the optimal treatment, which can provide definitive cure.

REFERENCES

1. Pohl H, Sirovich B, Welch HG. Esophageal adenocarcinoma incidence: are we reaching the peak? Cancer Epidemiol Biomarkers Prev 2010;19(6):1468–70.
2. Siegel R, Naishadham D, Jemal A. Cancer statistics, 2012. CA Cancer J Clin 2012;62(1):10–29.
3. Jankowski JA, Wright NA, Meltzer SJ, et al. Molecular evolution of the metaplasia-dysplasia-adenocarcinoma sequence in the esophagus. Am J Pathol 1999;154(4):965–73.
4. Werner M, Mueller J, Walch A, et al. The molecular pathology of Barrett's esophagus. Histol Histopathol 1999;14(2):553–9.
5. Collard JM. High-grade dysplasia in Barrett's esophagus. The case for esophagectomy. Chest Surg Clin N Am 2002;12(1):77–92.
6. Falk GW, Rice TW, Goldblum JR, et al. Jumbo biopsy forceps protocol still misses unsuspected cancer in Barrett's esophagus with high-grade dysplasia. Gastrointest Endosc 1999;49(2):170–6.
7. Birkmeyer JD, Siewers AE, Finlayson EV, et al. Hospital volume and surgical mortality in the United States. N Engl J Med 2002;346(15):1128–37.
8. Orringer MB, Marshall B, Chang AC, et al. Two thousand transhiatal esophagectomies: changing trends, lessons learned. Ann Surg 2007;246(3):363–72 [discussion: 372–4].
9. Oh DS, Hagen JA, Chandrasoma PT, et al. Clinical biology and surgical therapy of intramucosal adenocarcinoma of the esophagus. J Am Coll Surg 2006;203(2):152–61.
10. Rice TW, Blackstone EH, Adelstein DJ, et al. Role of clinically determined depth of tumor invasion in the treatment of esophageal carcinoma. J Thorac Cardiovasc Surg 2003;125(5):1091–102.
11. Rice TW, Zuccaro G Jr, Adelstein DJ, et al. Esophageal carcinoma: depth of tumor invasion is predictive of regional lymph node status. Ann Thorac Surg 1998;65(3):787–92.
12. Levine DS, Haggitt RC, Blount PL, et al. An endoscopic biopsy protocol can differentiate high-grade dysplasia from early adenocarcinoma in Barrett's esophagus. Gastroenterology 1993;105(1):40–50.
13. Schnell TG, Sontag SJ, Chejfec G, et al. Long-term nonsurgical management of Barrett's esophagus with high-grade dysplasia. Gastroenterology 2001;120(7):1607–19.
14. Pech O, Behrens A, May A, et al. Long-term results and risk factor analysis for recurrence after curative endoscopic therapy in 349 patients with high-grade intraepithelial neoplasia and mucosal adenocarcinoma in Barrett's oesophagus. Gut 2008;57(9):1200–6.
15. Pech O, Bollschweiler E, Manner H, et al. Comparison between endoscopic and surgical resection of mucosal esophageal adenocarcinoma in Barrett's esophagus at two high-volume centers. Ann Surg 2011;254(1):67–72.
16. Wang KK, Sampliner RE. Updated guidelines 2008 for the diagnosis, surveillance and therapy of Barrett's esophagus. Am J Gastroenterol 2008;103(3):788–97.
17. Levine DS, Blount PL, Rudolph RE, et al. Safety of a systematic endoscopic biopsy protocol in patients with Barrett's esophagus. Am J Gastroenterol 2000;95(5):1152–7.
18. Ormsby AH, Petras RE, Henricks WH, et al. Observer variation in the diagnosis of superficial oesophageal adenocarcinoma. Gut 2002;51(5):671–6.
19. Reid BJ, Levine DS, Longton G, et al. Predictors of progression to cancer in Barrett's esophagus: baseline histology and flow cytometry identify

low- and high-risk patient subsets. Am J Gastroen-terol 2000;95(7):1669–76.

20. Puli SR, Reddy JB, Bechtold ML, et al. Staging ac-curacy of esophageal cancer by endoscopic ultra-sound: a meta-analysis and systematic review. World J Gastroenterol 2008;14(10):1479–90.

21. Chemaly M, Scalone O, Durivage G, et al. Miniprobe EUS in the pretherapeutic assessment of early esophageal neoplasia. Endoscopy 2008; 40(1):2–6.

22. Dunbar KB, Spechler SJ. The risk of lymph-node metastases in patients with high-grade dysplasia or intramucosal carcinoma in Barrett's esophagus: a systematic review. Am J Gastroenterol 2012; 107(6):850–62 [quiz: 863].

23. Buttar NS, Wang KK, Sebo TJ, et al. Extent of high-grade dysplasia in Barrett's esophagus correlates with risk of adenocarcinoma. Gastroenterology 2001;120(7):1630–9.

24. Weston AP, Sharma P, Topalovski M, et al. Long-term follow-up of Barrett's high-grade dysplasia. Am J Gastroenterol 2000;95(8):1888–93.

25. Bolton WD, Hofstetter WL, Francis AM, et al. Impact of tumor length on long-term survival of pT1 esophageal adenocarcinoma. J Thorac Cardi-ovasc Surg 2009;138(4):831–6.

26. Ell C, May A, Pech O, et al. Curative endoscopic resection of early esophageal adenocarcinomas (Barrett's cancer). Gastrointest Endosc 2007; 65(1):3–10.

27. Pech O, May A, Gossner L, et al. Curative endo-scopic therapy in patients with early esophageal squamous-cell carcinoma or high-grade intraepi-thelial neoplasia. Endoscopy 2007;39(1):30–5.

28. Stein HJ, Feith M, Bruecher BL, et al. Early esoph-ageal cancer: pattern of lymphatic spread and prognostic factors for long-term survival after surgi-cal resection. Ann Surg 2005;242(4):566–73 [dis-cussion: 573–5].

29. Hirota WK, Zuckerman MJ, Adler DG, et al. ASGE guideline: the role of endoscopy in the surveillance of premalignant conditions of the upper GI tract. Gastrointest Endosc 2006;63(4):570–80.

30. Chang EY, Morris CD, Seltman AK, et al. The effect of antireflux surgery on esophageal carcinogenesis in patients with barrett esophagus: a systematic re-view. Ann Surg 2007;246(1):11–21.

31. Rice TW. Pro: esophagectomy is the treatment of choice for high-grade dysplasia in Barrett's esoph-agus. Am J Gastroenterol 2006;101(10):2177–9.

32. Sepesi B, Watson TJ, Zhou D, et al. Are endoscopic therapies appropriate for superficial submucosal esophageal adenocarcinoma? An analysis of esophagectomy specimens. J Am Coll Surg 2010;210(4):418–27.

33. Gockel I, Sgourakis G, Lyros O, et al. Risk of lymph node metastasis in submucosal esophageal cancer: a review of surgically resected patients. Expert Rev Gastroenterol Hepatol 2011;5(3): 371–84.

34. Manner H, Pech O, Heldmann Y, et al. Efficacy, safety, and long-term results of endoscopic treat-ment for early-stage adenocarcinoma of the esoph-agus with low-risk sm1 invasion. Clin Gastroenterol Hepatol 2013;11(6):630–5.

35. Westerterp M, Koppert LB, Buskens CJ, et al. Outcome of surgical treatment for early adenocar-cinoma of the esophagus or gastro-esophageal junction. Virchows Arch 2005;446(5):497–504.

36. Zemler B, May A, Ell C, et al. Early Barrett's carci-noma: the depth of infiltration of the tumour corre-lates with the degree of differentiation, the incidence of lymphatic vessel and venous invasion. Virchows Arch 2010;456(6):609–14.

37. Burmeister BH, Smithers BM, Gebski V, et al. Sur-gery alone versus chemoradiotherapy followed by surgery for resectable cancer of the oesophagus: a randomised controlled phase III trial. Lancet On-col 2005;6(9):659–68.

38. Tepper J, Krasna MJ, Niedzwiecki D, et al. Phase III trial of trimodality therapy with cisplatin, fluoro-uracil, radiotherapy, and surgery compared with surgery alone for esophageal cancer: CALGB 9781. J Clin Oncol 2008;26(7):1086–92.

39. Urba SG, Orringer MB, Turrisi A, et al. Randomized trial of preoperative chemoradiation versus surgery alone in patients with locoregional esophageal car-cinoma. J Clin Oncol 2001;19(2):305–13.

40. Walsh TN, Noonan N, Hollywood D, et al. A comparison of multimodal therapy and surgery for esophageal adenocarcinoma. N Engl J Med 1996;335(7):462–7.

41. van Hagen P, Hulshof MC, van Lanschot JJ, et al. Preoperative chemoradiotherapy for esophageal or junctional cancer. N Engl J Med 2012;366(22): 2074–84.

42. Sjoquist KM, Burmeister BH, Smithers BM, et al. Survival after neoadjuvant chemotherapy or che-moradiotherapy for resectable oesophageal carci-noma: an updated meta-analysis. Lancet Oncol 2011;12(7):681–92.

43. Fok M, Sham JS, Choy D, et al. Postoperative radiotherapy for carcinoma of the esophagus: a prospective, randomized controlled study. Surgery 1993;113(2):138–47.

44. Zieren HU, Muller JM, Jacobi CA, et al. Adjuvant postoperative radiation therapy after curative resection of squamous cell carcinoma of the thoracic esophagus: a prospective randomized study. World J Surg 1995;19(3):444–9.

45. A comparison of chemotherapy and radiotherapy as adjuvant treatment to surgery for esophageal carcinoma. Japanese Esophageal Oncology Group. Chest 1993;104(1):203–7.

46. Macdonald JS, Smalley SR, Benedetti J, et al. Chemoradiotherapy after surgery compared with surgery alone for adenocarcinoma of the stomach or gastroesophageal junction. N Engl J Med 2001; 345(10):725–30.

47. Gibson MK, Abraham SC, Wu TT, et al. Epidermal growth factor receptor, p53 mutation, and pathological response predict survival in patients with locally advanced esophageal cancer treated with preoperative chemoradiotherapy. Clin Cancer Res 2003;9(17):6461–8.

48. Safran H, DiPetrillo T, Nadeem A, et al. Trastuzumab, paclitaxel, cisplatin, and radiation for adenocarcinoma of the esophagus: a phase I study. Cancer Invest 2004;22(5):670–7.

49. Gorski DH, Beckett MA, Jaskowiak NT, et al. Blockage of the vascular endothelial growth factor stress response increases the antitumor effects of ionizing radiation. Cancer Res 1999;59(14): 3374–8.

50. Cooper JS, Guo MD, Herskovic A, et al. Chemoradiotherapy of locally advanced esophageal cancer: long-term follow-up of a prospective randomized trial (RTOG 85-01). Radiation Therapy Oncology Group. JAMA 1999;281(17):1623–7.

51. Herskovic A, Martz K, al-Sarraf M, et al. Combined chemotherapy and radiotherapy compared with radiotherapy alone in patients with cancer of the esophagus. N Engl J Med 1992;326(24): 1593–8.

Endoscopic Management of Barrett's Esophagus with High-Grade Dysplasia and Early-Stage Esophageal Adenocarcinoma

Marta L. Davila, MD[a],*, Wayne L. Hofstetter, MD[b]

KEYWORDS

- Intestinal metaplasia • Dysplasia • Radiofrequency ablation • Cryotherapy
- Endoscopic mucosal resection • Esophagectomy

KEY POINTS

- Endoscopic therapies have been shown to be effective and safe in the treatment of patients with Barrett's esophagus–high-grade dysplasia (BE-HGD) and early esophageal cancer while preserving the esophagus.
- Patients with mucosal adenocarcinoma arising from BE can be effectively treated with a combination of endoscopic resection followed by ablation.
- Close surveillance of these patients is recommended after endoscopic therapy because of the risk of recurrence.
- Given the complexities in the evaluation and management of these patients, it is best to manage them with a multidisciplinary team in a tertiary referral center with expertise in esophageal diseases.

INTRODUCTION

In the United States, Barrett's esophagus (BE) is defined as the replacement of esophageal squamous mucosa by intestinal-type specialized columnar epithelium with goblet cells.[1] BE is believed to be the result of long-standing gastroesophageal reflux disease and is the most important risk factor and precursor for esophageal adenocarcinoma (EAC).[2–4]

In the past several decades, the incidence of and mortality from EAC have been increasing at an alarming rate in the United States and other Western countries.[5] It becomes, therefore, imperative that we make an early diagnosis and institute appropriate treatment in the hopes of improving survival. This article reviews the current endoscopic treatment options for BE with high-grade dysplasia and early EAC.

ENDOSCOPIC SURVEILLANCE OF BE

Patients with BE can, through a series of degenerative DNA pathways, progress from nondysplastic intestinal metaplasia to low-grade dysplasia (LGD), high-grade dysplasia (HGD), intramucosal

The authors have nothing to disclose.
[a] Department of Gastroenterology, Hepatology and Nutrition, The University of Texas MD Anderson Cancer Center, 1515 Holcombe Boulevard, Unit 146, Houston, TX 77030, USA; [b] Department of Thoracic and Cardiovascular Surgery, The University of Texas MD Anderson Cancer Center, 1400 Pressler Avenue, Unit 1489, Houston, TX 77030, USA
* Corresponding author.
E-mail address: mdavila@mdanderson.org

Thorac Surg Clin 23 (2013) 479–489
http://dx.doi.org/10.1016/j.thorsurg.2013.07.010
1547-4127/13/$ – see front matter © 2013 Elsevier Inc. All rights reserved.

carcinoma, and eventually to invasive EAC.[6] The purpose of surveillance of BE has been to detect dysplasia and early EAC. Although the benefit of surveillance has not been conclusively proved, multiple studies have shown that patients with EAC who were undergoing surveillance had a lower stage of disease and improved survival when compared with those not undergoing surveillance.[7,8] Although those studies could be prone to lead-time and length-time biases, a number of gastroenterological societies have developed surveillance guidelines under the assumption that the practice will reduce deaths.

Because the risk of EAC varies depending on the degree of dysplasia, surveillance guidelines also vary based on histology (**Table 1**). Patients with nondysplastic BE are advised to undergo endoscopic surveillance every 3 to 5 years.[9,10] A careful inspection of the Barrett's segment with white light high-resolution endoscopes remains the standard of care, with 4-quadrant biopsies taken every 2 cm (Seattle protocol). Any degree of dysplasia should be confirmed by an expert pathologist.[9–13] Moreover, any mucosal irregularities should be biopsied and submitted separately to pathology. Patients with low-grade dysplasia (LGD) should undergo esophagogastroduodenoscopy (EGD) in 6 months to confirm this diagnosis, and yearly thereafter, with 4-quadrant biopsies every 1 to 2 cm. Some experts advocate endoscopic treatment of LGD, given its unpredictable natural history, and increased risk of progression to cancer when confirmed by 2 expert pathologists.[9,10]

Patients with BE and confirmed HGD should not undergo surveillance but be referred for endoscopic treatment.[9–13] There are two reasons for this recommendation. First, the risk of progression from HGD to adenocarcinoma is high, ranging from 6% to 19% per year, assuming no therapeutic intervention takes place and there are no macroscopically visible lesions.[14,15] Second, there is a risk of concomitant adenocarcinoma in patients diagnosed with BE-HGD. Although older literature reported an approximately 40% risk of harboring invasive cancer in patients undergoing esophagectomy for BE-HGD, more recent literature suggests that the rate may be as low as 3% in the absence of visible lesions and 11% in patients with visible lesions.[16]

Patients with BE-HGD unfit or unwilling to undergo treatment should consider surveillance EGD every 3 months with 4-quadrant biopsies every 1 cm.[9–11]

DIAGNOSIS AND STAGING

A careful examination of the Barrett's segment is recommended using high-definition white light endoscopy. In fact, the longer the time spent inspecting the Barrett's segment, the higher the likelihood of detecting suspicious lesions. In a study by Gupta and colleagues,[17] 112 patients underwent endoscopic surveillance by 11 endoscopists. Endoscopists who had an average inspecting time longer than 1 minute per centimeter BE detected more suspicious lesions than those who spent a minute or less, and there was a trend toward higher detection of HGD/EAC.

The extent of BE should be described using standardized criteria, such as the Prague C and M classification.[18] These validated criteria include assessment of the circumferential (C)

Table 1
Surveillance guidelines for patients with BE based on recommendations from gastroenterological and surgical societies

Diagnosis	Recommendations
Nondysplastic BE	EGD every 3–5 y Four-quadrant biopsies every 2 cm
BE with low-grade dysplasia	Obtain review from an expert pathologist Follow-up EGD in 6 mo to confirm diagnosis If confirmed, surveillance EGD every year with 4-quadrant biopsies every 1–2 cm Consider endoscopic resection or ablation
BE with high-grade dysplasia	Obtain review from an expert pathologist Refer for endoscopic resection or ablation Consider EUS in selected cases If patient unfit or unwilling to undergo endoscopic treatment, perform EGD every 3 mo with 4-quadrant biopsies every 1 cm

Abbreviations: BE, Barrett's esophagus; EGD, esophagogastroduodenoscopy; EUS, endoscopic ultrasound.
Adapted from Refs.[9–13]

and maximum (M) extent of the endoscopically visualized BE segment, as well as endoscopic landmarks. Any visible lesions should be described according to the Paris endoscopic classification of superficial neoplastic lesions.[19] Lesions can be divided into 3 categories: protruding (0-I), nonprotruding and nonexcavated (0-II), and excavated (0-III). Type 0-II lesions are then subdivided into slightly elevated (0-IIa), flat (0-IIb), or depressed (0-IIc). This classification may help predict the extent of invasion into submucosa and therefore the choice between endoscopic or surgical treatment. Protruding (0-I), excavated (0-III), and nonprotruding depressed lesions (0-IIc) are associated with a higher risk of submucosal invasion. The lowest risk appears to be in completely flat lesions (0-IIb).[19]

Several recent imaging technologies, for example, chromoendoscopy, narrow-band imaging (Olympus TM, Olympus America, Center Valley, PA, USA), autofluorescence imaging, and confocal laser endomicroscopy, have become available for detailed visualization and characterization of mucosal and cellular architecture. Although these technologies may be helpful in guiding the performance of biopsies, their role is still not well defined in the routine surveillance of patients with BE.[9,18]

Although endoscopic ultrasound (EUS) is routinely used to estimate the depth and nodal status of a visible invasive EAC, it has a limited role in the evaluation of patients with BE-HGD and early EAC. Most experts do not recommend EUS in patients with a flat Barrett's segment and HGD detected by biopsy. In the evaluation of superficial lesions, the accuracy of EUS staging is modest at best. In a study comparing the accuracy of high-resolution endoscopy and high-resolution endoscopic ultrasonography using miniprobes, the sensitivity of EUS staging for mucosal tumors was 90% and for submucosal tumors 46%, and these were not significantly different from the sensitivity of high-resolution endoscopy in experienced hands.[20] In a systematic review by Young and colleagues[21] comparing EUS staging to endoscopic mucosal resection (EMR) or surgical pathology for T1 and T2 tumors, EUS correctly predicted the T stage of the target lesion with 67% accuracy (12 studies, n = 132). On the basis of the individual patient-level analysis, the accuracy of correct staging was only 56%. There are several factors that may explain the poor performance of EUS in the setting of Barrett-related early adenocarcinoma: wall thickening due to inflammation, presence of a duplicated muscularis mucosa, anatomic changes at the level of the gastroesophageal junction (GEJ)/cardia, and the endoscopist's experience.[21]

Nevertheless, EUS-guided fine-needle aspiration (FNA) may be considered in select cases in which there is a possibility of detecting malignant lymphadenopathy.[10] In a study of 25 patients referred for EUS evaluation (12 diagnosed with BE-HGD and 13 with intramucosal adenocarcinoma), 5 patients were found to have submucosal involvement and 7 patients were found to have suspicious lymphadenopathy. FNA confirmed malignancy in 5 of the 7 patients. Based on these results, 5 patients (20%) were found to be unsuitable candidates for endoscopic therapy.[22] Studies like this one highlight the importance of a careful approach to individual patients with BE and mucosal lesions.

EMR has emerged as a diagnostic and therapeutic tool for patients with BE-related early adenocarcinoma.[9–13] EMR involves local snare excision of lesions by a variety of different techniques, including the popular cap-and-band ligation techniques. EMR allows for removal of mucosal and submucosal lesions and is superior to EUS for the assessment of local T status (depth of invasion). EMR can result in a change in pathologic diagnosis in 30% to 49% of cases.[23,24] In a prospective study of 75 patients with biopsy-proven HGD or early cancer, EMR histology resulted in altered grading or staging in 48% of patients (downgrading in 28% and upgrading in 20%).[23] In another study of 293 EMR procedures for focal lesions, the final histology led to a change in diagnosis in 49% of cases, and a change in treatment in 30%.[24]

In summary, optimal staging is key in the management of BE-associated mucosal lesions. Mucosal adenocarcinomas are associated with very low rates of lymph node metastases (<3%) and can be managed endoscopically,[25] whereas tumors invading the submucosa have a substantial risk of lymph node metastases (in excess of 20%) and should be referred for esophagectomy.[26]

ENDOSCOPIC TREATMENT

Endoscopic therapy can be divided into therapies that ablate or destroy tissue and therapies that resect tissue. Ablation therapies do not provide a pathologic specimen for examination and are considered suboptimal to resection therapies. However, ablation therapies can be applied to larger surface areas and to lesion locations that may not be amenable to resection. Ablation therapies include photodynamic therapy, thermal laser, APC (argon plasma coagulation), multipolar electrocoagulation, radiofrequency ablation (RFA), and cryoablation. Of those, RFA and cryoablation have recently increased in popularity, given their effectiveness, ease of use, and low risk of serious adverse effects.

RADIOFREQUENCY ABLATION

RFA (Covidien, Sunnyvale, CA) is a system that delivers high energy to the esophageal mucosa to achieve tissue destruction. The system generator is capable of delivering 10 to 12 J at a setting of 40 W/cm^2. The depth of ablation is between 500 and 1000 μm. There are 2 energy delivery systems available: a 3-cm-long balloon ablation catheter (HALO 360) intended to treat long-segment circumferential BE, and an endoscope-mounted targeted device (HALO 90, HALO 60, HALO ULTRA) to treat short segments and BE islands and tongues (**Fig. 1**). The technique involves mucosal ablation under endoscopic guidance followed by removal of the adhered white coagulum in the ablated area followed by repeat treatment of the same area, all within one endoscopic session. Multiple endoscopic treatments may be required depending on the length of the Barrett's segment and the tissue response. Treatment is usually performed about every 2 months.

In the past several years, multiple studies have demonstrated the efficacy, safety, and durability of RFA to treat dysplastic and nondysplastic BE.[15,27–29] In a multicenter study, 127 patients with dysplastic BE were randomly assigned in a 2:1 ratio to receive either RFA or sham procedure[15]; 84 patients were randomized to the RFA treatment group: 42 patients had HGD and 42 had LGD. On average, patients received 3.5 treatments. Among patients with HGD, complete eradication of dysplasia (CE-D) occurred in 81% of patients assigned to the ablation group as compared with 19% of those assigned to the control group (P<.001). Among patients with LGD, CE-D occurred in 90.5% of patients in the treatment arm, as compared with 22.7% of those assigned to the control group (P<.001). Overall, 77.4% of patients in the RFA group had complete eradication of intestinal metaplasia (CE-IM) compared with 2.3% of those in the control group (P<.001). Progression from HGD to cancer occurred in 4 of 21 patients in the control group and in only 1 of 42 patients in the RFA-treated group (P = .045). After this study was published, patients in the control group were offered ablation treatment and were followed for a mean time of 3.05 years.[27] In total, 119 patients received RFA treatment. At 2 years, among subjects with initial BE-HGD, there was CE-D in 93% and CE-IM in 89%. At 3 years, CE-D was reported in 98% of patients and CE-IM in 91%, but only 56 patients completed the study. The annual rate of progression to EAC among those treated with RFA was 0.55% per patient per year.[27]

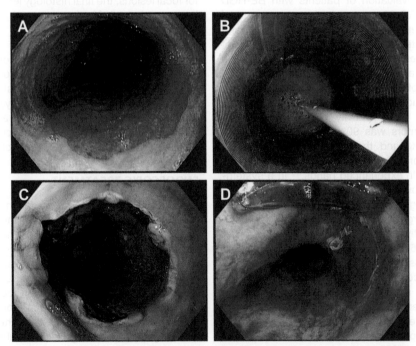

Fig. 1. (*A*) Endoscopic appearance of long-segment circumferential BE. (*B*) Endoscopic view of BE treated with the HALO 360 balloon electrode. (*C*) Endoscopic appearance after balloon treatment. (*D*) Treatment of a Barrett's island with the HALO 90 device.

A nonrandomized US multicenter registry study of circumferential RFA in 142 patients with HGD revealed similar results, with CE-HGD reported in 90% of patients and CE-IM in 54% at 12-month follow-up.[28] RFA treatment has also been found effective when performed in community practices. A multicenter registry conducted in 4 community-based gastroenterology practices reported the results of RFA treatment in 429 patients (91 patients with dysplastic BE). At a median follow-up of 20 months, CR-IM was achieved in 77% of patients with 100% achieving CE-D.[30]

RFA is safe and well tolerated. The most common complications reported include chest pain lasting less than 1 week, strictures requiring dilation (6%–8%), and gastrointestinal hemorrhage (1%).[15,31]

Subsquamous intestinal metaplasia (SSIM) or the presence of intestinal metaplasia beneath overlying squamous epithelium (so called "buried glands") has been reported following all ablative techniques, including photodynamic therapy, APC, and multipolar electrocoagulation. The main concern with SSIM is that it cannot be detected by endoscopic visual examination. Studies examining the prevalence of SSIM following RFA treatment indicate that RFA might decrease the prevalence of SSIM. In the only randomized sham-controlled trial of RFA for dysplastic BE,

25.2% of subjects were reported to have SSIM before ablation. Among patients treated with RFA, the prevalence of SSIM decreased to 5.1% after 12 months and 3.8% after 24 months.[15,27] Alternatively, SSIM was noted in 40% of patients randomized to sham procedure at 12-month follow-up.[15] In a prospective multicenter study of patients with nondysplastic BE treated with RFA, biopsy specimens obtained from 50 patients at 5-year follow-up revealed no evidence of SSIM.[29]

Following RFA treatment, BE (both dysplastic and nondysplastic) can recur, which means patients need to continue endoscopic surveillance following treatment. Recurrence rates at 1 year range from 5% to 25%.[32,33] No specific clinical characteristics have been associated with disease recurrence, although one study found that baseline BE length was significantly longer in those who developed recurrence.[32] Currently, there are no consensus recommendations regarding surveillance interval in patients after ablation. Some experts recommend surveillance endoscopy every 3 months for the first year, every 6 months for the second year, and then annually.[34]

CRYOTHERAPY

Cryotherapy is a noncontact ablative technique that causes tissue destruction by using cycles of rapid freezing and slow thawing (**Fig. 2**).[35] Two

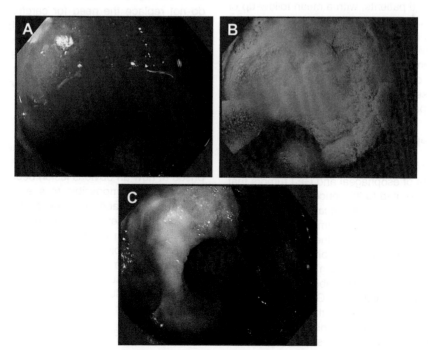

Fig. 2. (*A*) Endoscopic appearance of a Barrett's island. (*B*) Cryoablation treatment. (*C*) Thawing noted immediately after treatment with cryoablation.

devices are commercially available for endoscopic spray cryotherapy: one using liquid nitrogen, the other carbon dioxide. The technique involves advancing a decompression tube into the stomach to remove excess gas. A spray catheter is then advanced through the working channel of the endoscope and either liquid nitrogen or carbon dioxide is applied to the targeted area. Two to 3 cm of BE can be treated while covering about one-third or one-half of the luminal circumference. Multiple areas can be treated in one endoscopic session. On average, 3 to 4 endoscopies are needed to completely ablate a long-segment BE and the procedures can be performed about every 6 to 8 weeks.

There are no randomized controlled studies assessing the efficacy of cryotherapy in the treatment of dysplastic BE. In a multicenter retrospective study[36] of liquid nitrogen in patients with BE-HGD, 97% of patients had complete eradication of HGD and 87% had complete eradication of all dysplasia; 57% of patients had CE-IM at a mean follow-up of 10.5 months. The most common adverse events reported included strictures in 3%, which responded to endoscopic dilation, and chest pain in 2%, managed on an outpatient basis. A multicenter retrospective study of liquid nitrogen for esophageal cancer was published in 2010.[37] Complete eradication of T1a tumors occurred in 18 (75%) of 24 patients. For T1b (submucosal) tumors, complete eradication was seen in 4 (60%) of 6 patients, with a mean follow-up of 11.8 months.

There are no studies comparing cryotherapy to other ablative therapies and specific recommendations cannot be made regarding when to use cryotherapy over RFA. Among experts, cryotherapy has been used in patients who have failed RFA or to treat BE patients in the setting of strictures.

ENDOSCOPIC RESECTION

EMR is indicated in the staging workup and potential treatment of esophageal and GEJ tumors that appear to be limited to the mucosal or superficial submucosal layer.[38–41] Historically, the procedure gained acceptance in the treatment of polyps and early-staged cancers within the colon, but was later translated to use in esophageal squamous cell carcinoma, mainly in Asian medical centers. Since then, excellent results published by clinically active groups in Wiesbaden, Germany, and the Netherlands have encouraged the use of this modality for patients with esophageal and GEJ adenocarcinoma treated in Western centers.[38–42] Amenable lesions must be small enough to be completely resected endoscopically, with the lowest-risk lesions being smaller than 2 cm in maximal dimension.

The critical steps in the procedure involve the following (**Fig. 3**):

1. Identification of the lesion

When a target can be identified, one is more likely to completely remove the at-risk mucosa and index lesion (ie, cancerous or HGD) while avoiding the removal of too much mucosa, which may result in higher than necessary postprocedural complications, such as stricture, bleeding, or perforation. Endoscopists must be experienced at detecting the presence and severity of esophageal mucosal abnormality based on what is visualized through the endoscope. The equipment used for the procedure affects the clinician's ability to identify significant pathology and is critical to the outcome of endoscopic therapy. High-definition equipment is mandatory. Endoscopists must also be prepared to spend many minutes visualizing the entire circumference of the esophagus in areas of suspected pathology. Particular focus on the GEJ and cardia is warranted, as these are areas that are difficult to visualize because they can be poorly distended, are often angled or herniated, and have high incidences of tumor occurrence and recurrence. High-resolution white light and some form of chromoendoscopy, either filtered light or vital stains, allow the endoscopist to better visualize areas of abnormal mucosa, but they do not replace the need for careful observation over the entire area of suspicion. Experimental methods, such as autofluorescence or confocal microscopy, have been used to identify lesions that are difficult to see with standard endoscopy but have not gained traction in routine clinical settings thus far.

2. Outline the area of resection

Before beginning the resection, the area to be removed must be marked. We are frequently surprised at how an obvious lesion becomes difficult or all together impossible to see once a scope with a cap is placed into the esophagus, which obstructs our view. Marking the target area to include a margin of normal mucosa will help to avoid an incomplete resection. The endoscopist may also choose to place marks (cautery, ink, or clips) on the tissue immediately before resection to orient the tissue margins for the clinician and pathologist.

3. Perform the resection

Multiple methods of EMR or endoscopic submucosal dissection (ESD) are currently used.

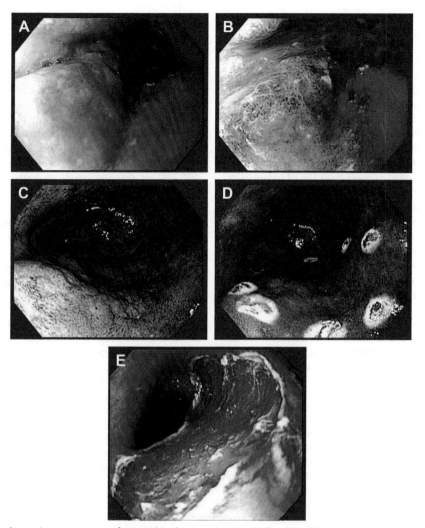

Fig. 3. (*A*) Endoscopic appearance of an early adenocarcinoma at the GEJ. (*B*) Appearance under narrow-band imaging (Olympus). (*C, D*) Cautery marks the margins of resection. (*E*) Appearance after resection.

Facile methods for EMR involve a cap-and-snare technique with or without a rubber band to create a suction polyp followed by a cauterized snare to resect down to the submucosal level while simultaneously achieving hemostasis. Smaller lesions and selected lesions that are up to 2 cm can be removed entirely en bloc with suction cap techniques. However, when larger lesions are approached with an EMR-cap technique they frequently require "piecemeal" resection, where the lesion is removed by multiple applications of the cap and snare to include overlapping areas, ultimately resulting in a complete resection.[42] On the other hand, ESD is more likely to achieve an en bloc resection for larger or deeper lesions but it is technically more difficult and results in more frequent complications, such as perforation or bleeding. For this reason, it is performed only in selected centers where specialized training has been performed.

4. Postresection management

Postresection management is often performed with the help of sedation; anesthesia support is optimal where available, but not critical. Patients are transferred to a recovery unit for an hour or so and then discharged home the same day, unless there are comorbidities or complications that mandate otherwise. We typically allow liquids the first day, soft foods for a few days afterward, and liberalization of diet when symptoms allow. Patients (and family accompanying) need to be educated on expected outcomes and potential signs of complications before the procedure; reiteration after the procedure is valuable. Written educational instructions are also extremely helpful.

Expected short-term outcomes include chest discomfort and odynophagia for a few days after resection, so we provide a compound prescription that includes sucralfate and a local anesthetic to alleviate these symptoms. Mild to moderate dysphagia can also be a frequent complaint associated with healing of the iatrogenic ulcer, but most often subsides after 6 to 8 weeks.

Typical complications are similar to other routine upper endoscopic procedures, with the most frequent event being aspiration. Specific to EMR, perforation is seen in fewer than 1% of cases using most cap techniques. This is in contrast to reports of perforation in upward of 40% for aggressive ESD procedures. However, almost all perforations, including those associated with ESD, can be handled nonoperatively. Bleeding risk is 2% to 3% for EMR. Stricture may occur and this depends on previous pathology in the individual patient and the amount of circumference removed at the time of resection. Removing more than 50% circumference significantly increases the risk of stricture, but complete circumferential resections can be performed. We typically like to stage procedures that will require circumferential resections into several episodes.

5. Interpretation of pathology

Lesions that are treated successfully with EMR are most often limited to the mucosa or superficial submucosa and have been completely resected. Submucosal invasion increases the risk of lymph node invasion and/or cancer-related events of recurrence or death. Lymphovascular invasion (LVI) is the most important prognostic determinant of outcome for resected early-stage cancer.[41,43] Typical risk of nodal involvement increases from 2% to 3% for a T1a lesion without LVI to 60%+ for T1b lesions with LVI.[25,41,43] Size of tumor and differentiation have been shown to be independent prognostic variables in some studies, where lesions smaller than 2 cm and well to moderately differentiated are less likely to harbor concurrent adenopathy.[39,41]

6. Follow-up

Most patients who are treated for HGD and/or mucosal carcinoma will require ablation to decrease the incidence of metachronous lesions or recurrence. This is discussed in detail later in this article. There are no established guidelines regarding the frequency of follow-up endoscopy or need for cross-sectional imaging of patients treated endoscopically for HGD or early carcinoma of the esophagus/GEJ. Based on surgical literature, it is assumed that recurrence will be recognized most often within the first 2 years after therapy, but this assumes close clinical follow-up. It has been our practice to perform endoscopy every 2 to 3 months while in the process of ablating residual metaplasia/dysplasia, followed by increasing intervals between procedures depending on the individual findings. The need for cross-sectional imaging is debated in small T1a lesions, given the low risk of regional or distant metastasis, and it is not at all indicated for patients with dysplasia only. Patients at higher risk for regional and distant disease, such as those with deeper or larger lesions, or those patients with LVI who have opted for endoscopic treatment alone based on preference or risk for esophageal resection, undergo imaging every 4 to 6 months in our clinic.

MULTIMODALITY THERAPY: COMBINING ENDOSCOPIC RESECTION WITH MUCOSAL ABLATION

After EMR has removed any mucosal cancer, the remaining BE segment should be eradicated even in the absence of dysplasia.[12] If the remaining BE segment is left untreated, the risk of metachronous lesions may be as high as 30%.[44] A number of studies have evaluated the efficacy and safety of combining EMR with photodynamic therapy and Argon plasma coagulation. Since those ablative techniques have been largely abandoned, attention has now turned to RFA as the procedure of choice to eradicate residual intestinal metaplasia. Pouw and colleagues[45] reported their experience with 23 patients who underwent EMR for visible lesions; 16 patients had early cancer and 7 patients had BE-HGD. RFA was performed at least 6 weeks after the EMR. CE-neoplasia was achieved in 100% of patients (median follow-up 22 months) and CE-IM in 88% of patients.

In a US retrospective study of 65 patients treated with EMR and RFA for nodular disease, and 104 patients treated with RFA alone for flat BE, there were no significant differences in CE-D and CE-IM between the 2 groups. Furthermore, the complication rates were similar, including strictures, which occurred in 4.6% of patients in the EMR-before-RFA group and in 7.7% of patients in the RFA-only group.[46]

Combined EMR with RFA may be the preferred approach over stepwise radical endoscopic resection for the treatment of BE-HGD associated with early cancer. In a multicenter study from the Netherlands, patients with a BE segment of 5 cm or smaller containing HGD/early cancer were randomized to stepwise radical endoscopic resection (SSER) or endoscopic resection followed by RFA.

Both groups achieved excellent (>90%) comparable rates of CE-neoplasia and CE-IM; however, those in the SSER group developed a significantly higher number of strictures requiring endoscopic dilation (88% in the SSER group compared with 14% in the EMR-RFA group, P<.001).[47]

But how does endoscopic treatment compare with esophagectomy? A specialized center retrospective study compared endoscopic therapy performed in 40 patients (22 with HGD and 18 with intramucosal cancer) with esophagectomy in 61 patients (13 with HGD and 48 with intramucosal cancer). Endoscopic therapy consisted of 102 endoscopic resections and 79 ablations. There was no difference in survival between the 2 groups (94% at 3 years), but compared with esophagectomy, endoscopic therapy was associated with significantly lower morbidity (39% vs 0%, P<.0001).[48]

In summary, EMR followed by RFA is an effective treatment modality for early cancer arising in the setting of BE. However, these techniques are best performed at high-volume referral centers by experienced endoscopists. The outcomes may not apply to general practices.

SUMMARY

Endoscopic therapies have been shown to be effective and safe in the treatment of patients with BE-HGD and early esophageal cancer while preserving the esophagus. Patients with mucosal adenocarcinoma arising from BE can be effectively treated with a combination of endoscopic resection followed by ablation. Close surveillance of these patients is recommended after endoscopic therapy because of the risk of recurrence. Given the complexities in the evaluation and management of these patients, it is best to manage them by a multidisciplinary team in a tertiary referral center with expertise in esophageal diseases.

REFERENCES

1. Sampliner RE. Practice guidelines on the diagnosis, surveillance and therapy of Barrett's esophagus. Am J Gastroenterol 1998;93:1028–31.
2. Jung KW, Talley NJ, Romero Y, et al. Epidemiology and natural history of intestinal metaplasia of the gastroesophageal junction and Barrett's esophagus: a population-based study. Am J Gastroenterol 2011; 106:1447–55.
3. Solaymani-Dodaran M, Logan RF, West J, et al. Risk of oesophageal cancer in Barrett's oesophagus and gastro-oesophageal reflux. Gut 2004;53: 1070–4.
4. Hvid-Jensen F, Pedersen L, Drewes AM, et al. Incidence of adenocarcinoma among patients with Barrett's esophagus. N Engl J Med 2011;365:1375–83.
5. Hur C, Miller M, Kong CY, et al. Trends in esophageal adenocarcinoma incidence and mortality. Cancer 2013;119(6):1149–58.
6. Goldblum JR. Barrett's esophagus and Barrett's-related dysplasia. Mod Pathol 2003;16:316–24.
7. Corley DA, Levin TR, Habel LA, et al. Surveillance and survival in Barrett's adenocarcinoma: a population based study. Gastroenterology 2002;122: 633–40.
8. Fountoulakis A, Zafirellis K, Donlan K, et al. Effect of surveillance of Barrett's oesophagus on clinical outcome of oesophageal cancer. Br J Surg 2004; 91:997–1003.
9. Spechler SJ, Sharma P, Souza RF, et al. American Gastroenterological Association medical position statement on the management of Barrett's esophagus. Gastroenterology 2011;140:1084–91.
10. Evans JA, Early DS, Fukami N, et al. The role of endoscopy in Barrett's esophagus and other premalignant conditions of the esophagus. Gastrointest Endosc 2012;76:1087–94.
11. Wang KK, Sampliner RE. Updated guidelines 2008 for the diagnosis, surveillance and therapy of Barrett's esophagus. Am J Gastroenterol 2008;103: 788–97.
12. Bennett C, Vakil N, Bergman J, et al. Consensus statements for management of Barrett's dysplasia and early stage esophageal adenocarcinoma, based on a Delphi process. Gastroenterology 2012;143:336–46.
13. Fernando HC, Murthy SC, Hofstetter W, et al. The Society of Thoracic Surgeons practice guideline series: guidelines for the management of Barrett's esophagus with high-grade dysplasia. Ann Thorac Surg 2009;87:1993–2002.
14. Rastogi A, Puli S, El-Serag HB, et al. Incidence of esophageal adenocarcinoma in patients with Barrett's esophagus and high-grade dysplasia: a meta-analysis. Gastrointest Endosc 2008;67:394–8.
15. Shaheen NJ, Sharma P, Overholt BF, et al. Radiofrequency ablation in Barrett's esophagus with dysplasia. N Engl J Med 2009;360:2277–88.
16. Konda VJ, Ross AS, Ferguson MK, et al. Is the risk of concomitant invasive esophageal cancer in high-grade dysplasia in Barrett's esophagus overestimated? Clin Gastroenterol Hepatol 2008;6:159–64.
17. Gupta N, Gaddam S, Wani SB, et al. Longer inspection time is associated with increase detection of high-grade dysplasia and esophageal adenocarcinoma in Barrett's esophagus. Gastrointest Endosc 2012;76:531–8.
18. Panossian AM, Raimondo M, Wolfsen HC. State of the art in the endoscopic imaging and ablation of Barrett's esophagus. Dig Liver Dis 2011;43:365–73.

19. Endoscopic Classification Review Group. Update on the Paris classification of superficial neoplastic lesions in the digestive tract. Endoscopy 2005;37: 570–8.

20. May A, Günter E, Roth F, et al. Accuracy of staging in early oesophageal cancer using high resolution endoscopy and high resolution endosonography: a comparative, prospective, and blinded trial. Gut 2004;53:634–40.

21. Young PE, Gentry AB, Acosta RD, et al. Endoscopic ultrasound does not accurately stage early adenocarcinoma or high-grade dysplasia of the esophagus. Clin Gastroenterol Hepatol 2010;8: 1037–41.

22. Shami VM, Villaverde A, Stearns L, et al. Clinical impact of conventional endosonography and endoscopic ultrasound-guided fine needle aspiration in the assessment of patients with Barrett's esophagus and high-grade dysplasia or intramucosal carcinoma who have been referred for endoscopic ablation therapy. Endoscopy 2006;38:157–61.

23. Moss A, Bourke MJ, Hourigan LF, et al. Endoscopic resection for Barrett's high-grade dysplasia and early esophageal adenocarcinoma: an essential staging procedure with long-term therapeutic benefit. Am J Gastroenterol 2010;105:1276–83.

24. Peters FP, Brakenhoff KP, Curvers WL, et al. Histologic evaluation of resection specimens obtained at 293 endoscopic resections in Barrett's esophagus. Gastrointest Endosc 2008;67:604–9.

25. Dunbar KB, Spechler SJ. The risk of lymph-node metastases in patients with high-grade dysplasia or intramucosal carcinoma in Barrett's esophagus: a systematic review. Am J Gastroenterol 2012;107: 850–62.

26. Enestvedt BK, Ginsberg GG. Advances in endoluminal therapy for esophageal cancer. Gastrointest Endosc Clin N Am 2013;23:17–39.

27. Shaheen NJ, Overholt BF, Sampliner RE, et al. Durability of radiofrequency ablation in Barrett's esophagus with dysplasia. Gastroenterology 2011;141: 460–8.

28. Ganz RA, Overholt BF, Sharma VK, et al. Circumferential ablation of Barrett's esophagus that contains high-grade dysplasia: a U.S. multicenter registry. Gastrointest Endosc 2008;68:35–40.

29. Fleischer DE, Overholt BF, Sharma VK, et al. Endoscopic radiofrequency ablation for Barrett's esophagus: 5-year outcomes from a prospective multicenter trial. Endoscopy 2010;42:781–9.

30. Lyday WD, Corbett FS, Kuperman DA, et al. Radiofrequency ablation of Barrett's esophagus: outcomes of 429 patients from a multicenter community practice registry. Endoscopy 2010;42:272–8.

31. Bulsiewicz WJ, Kim HP, Dellon ES, et al. Safety and efficacy of endoscopic mucosal therapy with radiofrequency ablation for patients with neoplastic Barrett's esophagus. Clin Gastroenterol Hepatol 2013;11(6):636–42.

32. Vaccaro BJ, Gonzalez S, Poneros JM, et al. Detection of intestinal metaplasia after successful eradication of Barrett's esophagus with radiofrequency ablation. Dig Dis Sci 2011;56:1996–2000.

33. Orman ES, Kim HP, Bulsiewicz WJ, et al. Intestinal metaplasia recurs infrequently in patients successfully treated for Barrett's esophagus with radiofrequency ablation. Am J Gastroenterol 2013;108(2): 187–95.

34. Titi M, Overhiser A, Ulusarac O, et al. Development of subsquamous high-grade dysplasia and adenocarcinoma after successful radiofrequency ablation of Barrett's esophagus. Gastroenterology 2012; 143:564–6.

35. Greenwald BD, Dumot JA. Cryotherapy for Barrett's esophagus and esophageal cancer. Curr Opin Gastroenterol 2011;27:363–7.

36. Shaheen NJ, Greenwald BD, Peery AF, et al. Safety and efficacy of endoscopic spray cryotherapy for Barrett's esophagus with high-grade dysplasia. Gastrointest Endosc 2010;71:680–5.

37. Greenwald BD, Dumot JA, Abrams JA, et al. Endoscopic spray cryotherapy for esophageal cancer: safety and efficacy. Gastrointest Endosc 2010;71: 686–93.

38. Pech O, Bollschweiler E, Manner H, et al. Comparison between endoscopic and surgical resection of mucosal esophageal adenocarcinoma in Barrett's esophagus at two high-volume centers. Ann Surg 2011;254(1):67–72.

39. Pech O, Behrens A, May A, et al. Long-term results and risk factor analysis for recurrence after curative endoscopic therapy in 349 patients with high-grade intraepithelial neoplasia and mucosal adenocarcinoma in Barrett's oesophagus. Gut 2008;57(9): 1200–6.

40. Manner H, Pech O, Heldmann Y, et al. Efficacy, safety, and long-term results of endoscopic treatment for early-stage adenocarcinoma of the esophagus with low-risk sm1 invasion. Clin Gastroenterol Hepatol 2013;11(6):630–5.

41. Lee L, Ronellenfitsch U, Hofstetter WL, et al. Predicting lymph node metastases in early esophageal adenocarcinoma using a simple scoring system. J Am Coll Surg 2013;217(2):191–9.

42. Pouw RE, van Vilsteren FG, Peters FP, et al. Randomized trial on endoscopic resection-cap versus multiband mucosectomy for piecemeal endoscopic resection of early Barrett's neoplasia. Gastrointest Endosc 2011;74(1):35–43.

43. Alvarez Herrero L, Pouw RE, van Vilsteren FG, et al. Risk of lymph node metastasis associated with deeper invasion by early adenocarcinoma of the esophagus and cardia: study based on endoscopic resection specimens. Endoscopy 2010;42(12):1030–6.

44. May A, Gossner L, Pech O. Local endoscopic therapy for intraepithelial high-grade neoplasia and early adenocarcinoma in Barrett's esophagus: acute-phase and intermediate results of a new treatment approach. Eur J Gastroenterol Hepatol 2002;14: 1085–91.

45. Pouw RE, Wirths K, Eisendrath P, et al. Efficacy of radiofrequency ablation combined with endoscopic resection for Barrett's esophagus with early neoplasia. Clin Gastroenterol Hepatol 2010;8:23–9.

46. Kim HP, Bulsiewicz WJ, Cotton CC, et al. Focal endoscopic mucosal resection before radiofrequency ablation is equally effective and safe compared with radiofrequency ablation alone for the eradication of Barrett's esophagus with advanced neoplasia. Gastrointest Endosc 2012;76:733–9.

47. Van Vilsteren FG, Pouw RE, Seewald S, et al. Stepwise radical endoscopic resection versus radiofrequency ablation for Barrett's oesophagus with high-grade dysplasia or early cancer: a multicenter randomized trial. Gut 2011;60:765–73.

48. Zehetner J, DeMeester SR, Hagen JA, et al. Endoscopic resection and ablation versus esophagectomy for high-grade dysplasia and intramucosal adenocarcinoma. J Thorac Cardiovasc Surg 2011; 141:39–47.

Surgery for Esophageal Cancer
Goals of Resection and Optimizing Outcomes

Nabil Rizk, MD

KEYWORDS

- Radial margins • Proximal margins • Distal margins • Lymphadenectomy • Esophageal cancer

KEY POINTS

- The extent of lymphadenectomy should vary based on the risk of nodal metastases.
- Achieving an R-0 resection is an important component of an esophagectomy.
- Preoperative chemoradiation improves the likelihood of achieving an R-0 resection, whereas preoperative chemotherapy alone does not.

Determining what defines an adequate esophageal resection to optimize long-term outcomes in esophageal cancer is an elusive goal. The primary reason for this ambiguousness is the almost total lack of good quality prospective randomized surgical trials that examine this question adequately. Most available data are derived from small retrospective series typically representing single institution series and their treatment biases. A likely central reason for this lack of data is that there are strongly held opinions by clinicians regarding the oncologic benefits derived from an esophageal resection. For some, surgery is considered palliative only, and this nihilism is reflected in a minimalist surgical approach; alternatively, some consider surgical resection to be a dominant contributor to improved survival in the management of esophageal cancer, and for these advocates, the more radical the procedure, the greater the perceived benefit. The reality is, however, likely to be somewhere between these 2 extremes; there is likely a minimal standard that needs to be met to achieve optimal oncologic benefit from an operation, beyond which there is likely no additional marginal benefit. A second and equally important consideration in optimizing outcomes for surgery of the esophagus is the balance between increased short-term complications and oncologic outcome with increasingly radical surgeries.

The intent of this article is to identify the goals of an appropriate esophagectomy for cancer, essentially defining the targets that should be achieved from an operation. Clearly, these targets are not monolithic, but rather should reflect the variability of the underlying disease process, including different tumor stages, tumor location, and tumor type. Furthermore, these targets also need to be balanced with the different risks of surgery, realizing that with increasing radicality, there are increased risks. The 2 aspects of the surgical approach that have been associated with long-term outcomes and that will be reviewed in this article are the extent of lymphadenectomy, as measured by the number of nodes removed and the location of the nodes removed, and the ability to achieve disease free surgical margins, termed R-0 resections.

EXTENT OF LYMPHADENECTOMY

The extent of the lymphadenectomy needed in an esophagectomy is controversial. The argument primarily centers on the number of lymph node

Disclosures: The author has nothing to disclose.
Department of Surgery, Thoracic Service, Memorial Sloan-Kettering Cancer Center, 1275 York Avenue, C 883, New York, NY 10065, USA
E-mail address: rizkn@mskcc.org

Thorac Surg Clin 23 (2013) 491–498
http://dx.doi.org/10.1016/j.thorsurg.2013.07.009
1547-4127/13/$ – see front matter © 2013 Elsevier Inc. All rights reserved.

"fields" that need to be resected, as well as the minimum number of nodes that need to be removed. In fact, unlike most other malignancies, there is still the belief by some that, in esophageal cancer, beyond a complete primary tumor resection, a more extensive lymphadenectomy can result in improved survival. Despite this ongoing debate, the reality is that in the United States, this controversy is reserved primarily to the literature, because as in other malignancies such as gastric cancer or lung cancer, surgeons usually perform a minimal lymphadenectomy. This minimalist lymphadenectomy was documented prospectively in the Z0060 trial whereby the median number of nodes removed was 11, and only 36% of patients had 15 or more nodes removed.[1] Likewise, the retrospective Worldwide Esophageal Cancer Collaboration Data (WECC) study showed that only 41% of patients had 15 or more nodes removed.[2] This variability in extent of lymphadenectomy is pervasive even in the published literature, creating a situation whereby data regarding issues such as location of nodal metastases and likelihood of developing nodal metastases are not very reliable.

Likelihood of Nodal Metastases

The likelihood of developing nodal metastases is directly correlated with the depth of tumor invasion, and depth of invasion should therefore have an impact on the aggressiveness of the lymph node dissection. T1a tumors and superficial T1b tumors rarely metastasize to lymph nodes.[3] These data would argue then that a minimal to no lymphadenectomy should be needed in these patients, and that a procedure such as mucosal resection or transhiatal esophagectomy should be adequate treatment. Conversely, deeper submucosal tumors more frequently metastasize to lymph nodes, with some series showing a greater than 40% incidence of nodal disease.[3,4] This high likelihood of disease mandates a much more aggressive lymphadenectomy in these patients. Last, adequately resected T2 tumors are 60% to 80% likely[5,6] to contain nodal metastases, whereas greater than 80% of T3 tumors will have evidence of nodal disease.[5,6] There also seem to be some differences in the propensity to develop nodal metastases between squamous cell carcinomas and adenocarcinomas. Stein and co-workers[7] show that the likelihood to have nodal metastases was greater in mucosal squamous cell cancers compared with adenocarcinoma (7% vs 0%), as well as in submucosal tumors (36% vs 21%, respectively). This difference might have implications on tumor-specific success of local resection treatments in early stage cancers.

Location of Nodal Metastases

The most recent American Joint Committee on Cancer staging system categorizes all lymph nodes extending from the peri-esophageal cervical nodes down to the celiac axis as within the "zone" of regional disease.[8] Although many studies have shown that primary tumor location predisposes toward certain distribution patterns of nodal metastases, in reality there is sufficient variability in the potential sites on nodal spread that selecting nodal basins to resect based on the site of the primary tumor will invariably miss disease in some patients. The relevant question regarding this variability is whether a selective lymphadenectomy based on the site of the primary tumor is appropriate, or whether the variability of lymphatic spread needs to be addressed by removing all possible sites of disease. Proponents of selective lymphadenectomy point to data supporting the strong association between site of tumor origin and likely nodal drainage basins; in patients with disease beyond these usual sites, the assumption is that this indicates a burden of nodal disease representative of advanced stage disease.[9] Selective drainage implies that tumors in the upper esophagus tend to spread superiorly to the upper mediastinal and cervical regions first and are best managed by resection of these nodes, whereas lower esophageal and gastroesophageal tumors spread primarily to the upper abdominal and lower para-esophageal nodes, and mid-esophageal tumors spread bidirectionally.[10] Using this selective approach, for instance, Feith and colleagues[9] have shown that Siewert I tumors that arise below the level of the carina metastasize primarily to lower para-esophageal and upper abdominal nodes and rarely above the carina. Similarly, the study of Schröder and colleagues[11] of patterns of nodal metastases in Siewert I tumors showed that, when present, nodal metastases always have an intra-abdominal nodal component, with 25% having additional lower mediastinal disease, and only 10% of patients with nodal disease to the level of the carina. Likewise, others have shown that Siewert II and III tumors even more rarely metastasize to intrathoracic nodes,[12] and that therefore the focus of a lymphadenectomy in these tumors should be primarily on the intra-abdominal compartment, with limited inclusion of the lower mediastinal nodes.[13] One inconsistency of many practitioners of a selective lymphadenectomy, however, is that they often do not resect cervical and upper mediastinal nodes in mid-esophageal tumors (especially squamous cell cancers) despite the evidence supporting its benefits[14]; this raises the criticism that many who espouse selective lymphadenectomy in fact are not doing so consistently in mid-esophageal tumors.

What the selective approach to lymphadenectomies fails to address is the presence of unexpected drainage patterns and skip metastases. Several studies in which a thorough lymphadenectomy has been performed have shown a high incidence of skip metastases. Skip metastases have been well documented to occur by both in adenocarcinoma[5,6,15] with an incidence of about 30%, and up to 76% in squamous cell carcinoma.[10] Because of this variability as well as the belief in the benefits of a therapeutic lymphadenectomy, there are some who argue for routine 3-field lymphadenectomy for either all tumors[5,16] or for a subset of patients thought to be at higher risk for skip metastases, such as Siewert I adenocarcinoma with a moderate nodal burden.[6]

Describing the Extent of Lymphadenectomy

Lymphadenectomies during esophagectomies are most commonly divided into 3 fields. The first field is intra-abdominal and includes nodes on the lesser curvature of the stomach, nodes between the pancreas and the crura, and nodes along the hepatic, splenic, common hepatic, and left gastric arteries. These nodes are the most commonly involved lymph nodes in gastroesophageal junction tumors,[12,13] yet they tend to be the most frequently undersampled nodes by thoracic surgeons. The second field of lymph nodes is intrathoracic. These nodes are variously described as extending from either the carina down to the hiatus (most common description) or also including all superior mediastinal nodes up to the thoracic inlet including nodes along the right and left recurrent nerves.[5] The nodes from the second field are less commonly involved with disease than the first field in adenocarcinomas.[11,13] Although resection of the second field typically is performed using a right thoracotomy, the ability to resect the lower para-esophageal nodes via a thoracotomy is somewhat compromised due to difficulties in visualizing the region. A more effective retrieval method of these nodes is either with a minimally invasive approach or by a laparotomy and a radical transhiatal approach.[17] The classically described third field in an esophageal lymphadenectomy is resected via a cervical incision and includes the removal of nodes along both the recurrent nerves and the deep cervical nodes lateral and posterior to the common carotid sheath.[18] Some consider the superior mediastinal nodes to also be part of the third field.[6]

Another means of defining the extent of a lymphadenectomy is by quantifying the number of nodes that are removed. This descriptor adds a dimension of quality control to a lymphadenectomy because the number of nodes removed can reveal the aggressiveness of the lymphadenectomy, whereas the lymph node field description only describes the location of the nodes removed. On the other hand, using the number of nodes removed as a quality standard has its own limitations, including the fact that there is no control over which nodes are removed. Furthermore, quantifying the number of nodes removed can be subjective, partly dependent on how involved surgeons are at identifying the nodes for the pathologists, and partly dependent on the level of effort the pathologists make at counting the nodes. The most dependable description of a lymphadenectomy is to describe which fields were dissected as well as to provide the number of nodes removed.

Risks of Lymphadenectomy

The increased risks of a more extensive lymphadenectomy have been shown in several studies and are likely attributable to the additional exposure needed to perform it, the anatomic proximity of surrounding structures (thoracic duct, recurrent nerves, airway), and the additional operative time. A more thorough upper abdominal lymphadenectomy (D1 vs D2) has been shown in some randomized gastrectomy trials to be associated with increased morbidity and mortality.[19] Likewise, a 2-field lymphadenectomy generally requires an intrathoracic component to the procedure; if this is performed with a thoracotomy, there has clearly been shown to be an association with increased morbidity and mortality.[20] Furthermore, in performing a complete 2-field lymphadenectomy, the potential for a thoracic duct injury is greater than when a more limited lymphadenectomy is performed.[20] The added risks of a thoracotomy might be mitigated, however, by using a minimally invasive approach. Last, some studies have shown dramatically higher complication rates when removing the third field of nodes, with a significantly increased potential for unilateral and bilateral recurrent nerve injury; one randomized study had a greater than 50% tracheostomy incidence.[14] This reason and the preponderance of adenocarcinomas seen in the West are the most commonly cited reasons a third field lymphadenectomy is rarely performed.

Evidence Supporting a Lymphadenectomy

The evidence that the type and extent of lymphadenectomy is correlated with outcome is likely confounded by 2 important variables. The first is stage migration. Most of the data that support a correlation between the extent of a lymphadenectomy and outcome are retrospective, and therefore, cannot differentiate between stage migration or survival benefit. The second confounder is the fact that the various retrospective studies have varying distributions of pathologic stages, making comparisons of results difficult given the varying likelihood of metastatic nodal disease among different stages. Last, some retrospective studies also include patients who received preoperative therapy; in these patients it is difficult to account for nodal down-staging.

The most convincing evidence supporting the added benefit of extending a lymphadenectomy during an esophagectomy comes from the Hulscher trial.[17] In this well-controlled prospective randomized trial comparing an en-bloc esophagectomy, which included a complete lower mediastinal lymphadenectomy and a right paratracheal lymphadenectomy to a radical transhiatal esophagectomy, long-term follow-up showed that including a more thorough intrathoracic lymphadenectomy improved survival in patients with Siewert I tumors with 1 to 8 nodes involved with disease.[21] Even though this result was derived from an unplanned subset analysis, what makes the data more compelling is that they are consistent with the expectation that a lymphadenectomy should only be helpful if the patient is at risk for nodal disease or if the potential exists that the nodes removed represent all the possible disease sites (this would be less likely the more nodes are involved). This result is also consistent with the WECC retrospective study on the correlation between extent of lymphadenectomy and survival, as well as in the study by Schwarz and Smith.[22] The WECC study, unlike previous studies that supported a single minimal lymphadenectomy standard to optimize survival,[23,24] contained a sufficient number of patients to identify stage-dependent minimal lymphadenectomy standards.[2] Thus, patients at minimal to no risk of lymph nodal metastases (T1 tumors) derived no benefit from a more extensive lymphadenectomy, nor did patients with significant nodal disease ($\geq$7 nodes), whereas patients with a moderate risk for nodal metastases showed a graduated benefit from a more extensive lymphadenectomy as the risk and presence for nodal disease increased. These retrospective findings, although subject to the previously listed pitfalls, nevertheless seem to confirm the findings of the randomized trial.

Recommendations

Based on the available data, a reasonable approach in deciding the extent of a lymphadenectomy for esophageal cancer should incorporate the clinical stage and location of the disease, and the potential for nodal metastases, with the caveat that any benefit from a lymphadenectomy is due to stage migration, or from an actual survival benefit, or from both. Patients at very low risk (T1a, superficial T1b) likely do not need a lymphadenectomy, implying that a mucosal resection or a transhiatal esophagectomy would be an adequate surgical approach. Patients at moderate risk for nodal disease (deep T1b, T2) need a more extensive lymphadenectomy (15–20 nodes) and patients at highest risk (T3) need the most extensive lymphadenectomy (>30 nodes). With regard to which fields need to be resected, clearly the first and modified second (infra-azygous) are the most relevant for most adenocarcinomas and lower esophageal squamous cell cancers, and the second and potentially the third fields are the most relevant for mid-esophageal squamous cell carcinomas. More controversial are the removal of superior mediastinal nodes and possibly cervical nodes for Siewert I lesions as advocated by some, and limiting the lower mediastinal lymphadenectomy in Siewert III tumors. These 2 factors (number and location of nodes) should then dictate which surgical approaches should be considered.

RESECTION MARGIN
Definition

Resection margin (R-resection) refers to whether radial, proximal, or distal margins are grossly involved with disease (R-2), are completely uninvolved (R-0), or either have direct microscopic involvement at the margins as defined by the College of American Pathologists (R-1, College of American Pathologists criteria) or, as defined by the Royal College of Pathologists (RCP), have margins measured at less than 1 mm from the cut surface (R-1, RCP criteria).[25] These 2 definitions of an R-1 resection, while on the surface seeming to be insignificant, in fact can be associated with significant consequences if decisions regarding adjuvant radiation are based on a pathologic finding of an R-1 resection. In esophagectomies, there is also a separate distinction made between radial margins (the margins extending laterally from the esophageal wall and tumor), and the proximal (esophageal) and distal (gastric) margins. Most studies that refer to R-resection rates focus primarily on the radial margins. Proximal and distal margins are much less often involved with disease, although several specific issues deserve mention, including the extent of gastric resection needed in Siewert II and Siewert III cancers, the extent of proximal margin needed in squamous cell cancers, and the relevance of dysplasia and metaplasia at the proximal margin. Last, there is an important difficult management question that occasionally arises at the time of the operation or in the final pathology report, namely, what to do about a positive intraoperative margin.

Association with Outcome

Various studies have documented an association between R-resection and survival. A significant limitation in most of these data, however, is the inclusion of various proportions of patients at no risk of involved radial margins (anyone <T3), assuming an appropriate operation is performed. Furthermore, many of these studies fail to control for stage of disease in their analysis. The most convincing studies, namely those only including T3 tumors and that control for pathologic stage, do show an association between an R-1 resection and worse outcome. Using the College of American Pathologists criteria and controlling for depth of invasion, for instance, Deeter and colleagues[25] and Verhage and colleagues[26] show that survival is worse in R-1 resections. Others,[27–29] on the other hand, show that the RCP criteria are more relevant or predictive. Last, there are some who show that the involvement of radial margins is not relevant when controlling for stage[30] and rather serves as an indictor of more aggressive disease.

Operative Approach

Although the operative approach can have an impact on the ability to achieve an R-0 resection, optimization of various standard techniques can achieve fairly similar rates of R-0 resection among different operations. For instance, although one population-based retrospective study[31] suggested that a transhiatal esophagectomy is more often associated with R-1 resections, with a consequent impact on overall survival, the Hulscher trial clearly shows similar R-0 resection rates can be achieved when the standard transhiatal approach is extended to a "radical" transhiatal approach, wherein the lower mediastinum is able to be exposed to a much greater degree than in the standard transhiatal approach.[17] A radical transhiatal approach requires splitting of the diaphragm for better exposure. Likewise, when the intrathoracic component of an Ivor Lewis resection is extended to an en-bloc resection, R-0 resection rates as high as 90% are reported,[5] although these high rates are somewhat biased by the presence of some tumors less than T3 in the series. The extension to an en-bloc approach requires routine resection of the thoracic duct, the pericardium, and the contralateral pleura. In summary, various surgical approaches can achieve a greater likelihood of an R-0 resection; in theory, the more radical the approach, in which additional tissue planes are removed en bloc with the tumor, the more likely this can be achieved. Last, although proponents of the en-bloc approach claim that the improved R-0 resection rates are associated with a decreased incidence of local recurrences,[32] an alternate explanation for higher R-0 resection rates after an en-bloc esophagectomy other than attributing the benefits to resection of the thoracic duct, pericardium, and pleura, is that in mandating resection of these structures, a certain quality is guaranteed.

Impact of Induction Therapy

A consistent finding in the literature is that the addition of radiation to preoperative multimodality therapy increases the proportion of patients who achieve an R-0 resection relative to surgery alone. The recently published *Chemoradiotherapy for Oesophageal Cancer* trial confirms the findings from previous trials by showing that postchemoradiotherapy patients can achieve a 92% R-0 resection rate compared with 69% in those who undergo an operation only.[33] Likewise, consistently in the literature, chemotherapy alone does not increase the likelihood of an R-0 resection. This was shown by Kelsen and coworkers[34] in a prospective randomized neoadjuvant chemotherapy trial, whereby the R-0 resection rates were 59% after surgery only, and 62% after chemotherapy followed by surgery. One possible explanation why neoadjuvant chemoradiotherapy might be superior to chemotherapy only, therefore, is due to the improved R-0 resection rates. In fact, proponents of an en-bloc esophagectomy often claim that one reason they prefer neoadjuvant chemotherapy alone is that an en-bloc resection achieves similar R-0 resection rates as seen after neoadjuvant chemoradiation.

Gastric Margin and Siewert II/III Tumors

The management of tumors that straddle the gastroesophageal junction remains controversial. Some recommend a routine gastrectomy for any tumor with significant extension into the gastric cardia (Siewert II/III), partly because of concerns of recurrent disease in the gastric remnant, partly because of the belief that the nodal drainage is primarily intra-abdominal.[35] In these patients, the recommended surgical resection is a complete gastrectomy with minimal esophageal resection and lower para-esophageal lymphadenectomy, and a jejunal-esophageal anastomosis.[13] The concern with this approach is the potential compromise of the extent of the proximal margin.[36] Conversely, and especially in light of the new American Joint Committee on Cancer categorization of these tumors as esophageal cancers,[8] others think that these tumors should be managed with whichever approach is capable of best achieving an R-0 resection, using either a gastrectomy with a jejunal interposition, an esophagogastrectomy using the residual stomach as a conduit, or a gastrectomy and esophagectomy using the colon as a conduit.[37–40]

Proximal Esophageal Margins and Squamous Cell Cancer

Another area of controversy regarding margins is in esophageal squamous cell cancers. The concern in these cancers is the presence of either multifocal disease or proximal extension of submucosal disease beyond the main tumor mass, with the potential for persistent disease in the proximal esophageal remnant. Lam and coworkers[41] showed that the incidence of intramural spread beyond the primary tumor can occur both proximally and distally in up to 72% of cases, and up to 9 cm in distance. Tsutsui and colleagues[42] showed a similarly high incidence (up to 55%) and correlated the distance of spread to the depth of invasion of the primary tumor. This consideration prompts some to routinely recommend a complete esophagectomy in patients with esophageal squamous cell cancer, regardless of the proximal extent of the known tumor mass.

Dysplasia and Metaplasia at the Proximal Margin

One concern in Barrett's associated esophageal adenocarcinomas is the potential presence of dysplasia and/or metaplasia at the proximal margin. Clearly one goal of the resection needs to be resection of the esophagus proximal to involved sites; occasionally, however, technical concerns regarding conduit length and viability can limit the proximal extent of esophagus that can be resected. The data regarding the necessity of avoiding dysplastic or metaplastic proximal margins are virtually inexistent. However, with the availability of successful endoscopic treatments of dysplasia and metaplasia, it would seem that this concern should become less prominent.

A Positive Intraoperative Frozen Section Margin

A well-planned and executed operation should almost always be able to achieve proximal and distal margins that are uninvolved with disease (R-0 resection). Occasionally, however, one will encounter a situation intraoperatively of a "positive" microscopic margin (R-1 resection) with no easy recourse without significantly expanding the scope and risks of the operation. In these instances, the obvious question is, is it worth the added risk to achieve a negative intraoperative margin? The assumption in such a question needs to be that the operation was well planned and executed, and therefore, the involved margins were completely unexpected based on the clinical assessment of the extent and type of disease. Under these circumstances, the presence of an involved margin is frequently an indicator of more advanced underlying disease, and as with gastric cancers, the involved microscopic margin frequently becomes irrelevant prognostically.[43] Given the unavailability of detailed staging data during an operation, reconsideration on how to manage the margins can be made after the final pathologic information is available and a more accurate prognosis can be made.

Recommendations

Given the likely association between margins and survival, achieving an R-0 resection should be a major component of attempting to curatively treat patients with esophageal cancers. The radial margin is the most commonly involved margin in locally advanced (T3, T4) tumors. Minimizing this risk can be done either with the addition of preoperative chemoradiation or through a more aggressive radial resection, including an en-bloc resection if necessary. Proximal and distal margins are much less often involved, but there are specific issues that need to be taken into consideration to improve long-term survival. In tumors involving the gastroesophageal junction with significant gastric cardia involvement, a gastrectomy should be considered to achieve an R-0 resection, with the caveat that proximal margins are not compromised. Similarly, a total esophagectomy should be considered in squamous cell cancers because of the high potential for submucosal extension of disease. Last, in situations of appropriate surgical planning and execution, and an R-1 resection on frozen section, a reasonable approach would be to review the final pathology report first before extending the operation significantly; often in these situations, the long-term prognosis is sufficiently poor that a more aggressive local treatment is unwarranted.

REFERENCES

1. Veeramachaneni NK, Zoole JB, Decker PA, et al, American College of Surgeons Oncology Group

Z0060 Trial. Lymph node analysis in esophageal resection: American College of Surgeons Oncology Group Z0060 trial. Ann Thorac Surg 2008;86(2): 418–21 [discussion: 421].

2. Rizk NP, Ishwaran H, Rice TW, et al. Optimum lymphadenectomy for esophageal cancer. Ann Surg 2010;251(1):46–50.

3. Ancona E, Rampado S, Cassaro M, et al. Prediction of lymph node status in superficial esophageal carcinoma. Ann Surg Oncol 2008;15(11):3278–88.

4. Bollschweiler E, Baldus SE, Schröder W, et al. High rate of lymph-node metastasis in submucosal esophageal squamous-cell carcinomas and adenocarcinomas. Endoscopy 2006;38(2):149–56.

5. Lerut T, Nafteux P, Moons J, et al. Three-field lymphadenectomy for carcinoma of the esophagus and gastroesophageal junction in 174 R0 resections: impact on staging, disease-free survival, and outcome: a plea for adaptation of TNM classification in upper-half esophageal carcinoma. Ann Surg 2004;240(6):962–72 [discussion: 972–4].

6. Altorki N, Kent M, Ferrara C, et al. Three-field lymph node dissection for squamous cell and adenocarcinoma of the esophagus. Ann Surg 2002;236(2): 177–83.

7. Stein HJ, Feith M, Bruecher BL, et al. Early esophageal cancer: pattern of lymphatic spread and prognostic factors for long-term survival after surgical resection. Ann Surg 2005;242(4):566–73 [discussion: 573–5].

8. Edge SB, Byrd DR, Compton CC, et al, editors. AJCC cancer staging Manual. 7th edition. Springer; 2010.

9. Feith M, Stein HJ, Siewert JR. Pattern of lymphatic spread of Barrett's cancer. World J Surg 2003; 27(9):1052–7.

10. Chen J, Liu S, Pan J, et al. The pattern and prevalence of lymphatic spread in thoracic oesophageal squamous cell carcinoma. Eur J Cardiothorac Surg 2009;36(3):480–6.

11. Schröder W, Mönig SP, Baldus SE, et al. Frequency of nodal metastases to the upper mediastinum in Barrett's cancer. Ann Surg Oncol 2002; 9(8):807–11.

12. Fox MP, van Berkel V. Management of gastroesophageal junction tumors. Surg Clin North Am 2012; 92(5):1199–212.

13. Rüdiger Siewert J, Feith M, Werner M, et al. Adenocarcinoma of the esophagogastric junction: results of surgical therapy based on anatomical/topographic classification in 1,002 consecutive patients. Ann Surg 2000;232(3):353–61.

14. Nishihira T, Hirayama K, Mori S. A prospective randomized trial of extended cervical and superior mediastinal lymphadenectomy for carcinoma of the thoracic esophagus. Am J Surg 1998;175(1): 47–51.

15. Hosch SB, Stoecklein NH, Pichlmeier U, et al. Esophageal cancer: the mode of lymphatic tumor cell spread and its prognostic significance. J Clin Oncol 2001;19(7):1970–5.

16. Igaki H, Tachimori Y, Kato H. Improved survival for patients with upper and/or middle mediastinal lymph node metastasis of squamous cell carcinoma of the lower thoracic esophagus treated with 3-field dissection. Ann Surg 2004;239(4):483–90.

17. Hulscher JB, van Sandick JW, de Boer AG, et al. Extended transthoracic resection compared with limited transhiatal resection for adenocarcinoma of the esophagus. N Engl J Med 2002;347(21):1662–9.

18. Cense HA, van Eijck CH, Tilanus HW. New insights in the lymphatic spread of oesophageal cancer and its implications for the extent of surgical resection. Best Pract Res Clin Gastroenterol 2006;20(5): 893–906.

19. Bonenkamp JJ, Songun I, Hermans J, et al. Randomised comparison of morbidity after D1 and D2 dissection for gastric cancer in 996 Dutch patients. Lancet 1995;345:745–8.

20. Hulscher JB, Tijssen JG, Obertop H, et al. Transthoracic versus transhiatal resection for carcinoma of the esophagus: a meta-analysis. Ann Thorac Surg 2001;72(1):306–13.

21. Omloo JM, Lagarde SM, Hulscher JB, et al. Extended transthoracic resection compared with limited transhiatal resection for adenocarcinoma of the mid/distal esophagus: five-year survival of a randomized clinical trial. Ann Surg 2007;246(6): 992–1000 [discussion: 1000–1].

22. Schwarz RE, Smith DD. Clinical impact of lymphadenectomy extent in resectable esophageal cancer. J Gastrointest Surg 2007;11(11):1384–93 [discussion: 1393–4].

23. Rizk NP, Venkatraman E, Park B, et al. The prognostic importance of the number of involved nodes in esophageal cancer: implications for revisions of the American Joint Committee on Cancer Staging System. J Thorac Cardiovasc Surg 2006;132: 1374–81.

24. Peyre CG, Hagen JA, DeMeester SR, et al. The number of lymph nodes removed predicts survival in esophageal cancer: an International Study on the Impact of Extent of Surgical Resection. Ann Surg 2008;248:190–7.

25. Deeter M, Dorer R, Kuppusamy MK, et al. Assessment of criteria and clinical significance of circumferential resection margins in esophageal cancer. Arch Surg 2009;144(7):618–24.

26. Verhage RJ, Zandvoort HJ, ten Kate FJ, et al. How to define a positive circumferential resection margin in T3 adenocarcinoma of the esophagus. Am J Surg Pathol 2011;35(6):919–26.

27. Dexter SP, Sue-Ling H, McMahon MJ, et al. Circumferential resection margin involvement: an

independent predictor of survival following surgery for oesophageal cancer. Gut 2001;48(5):667–70.

28. Pultrum BB, Honing J, Smit JK, et al. A critical appraisal of circumferential resection margins in esophageal carcinoma. Ann Surg Oncol 2010; 17(3):812–20.

29. Rao VS, Yeung MM, Cooke J, et al. Comparison of circumferential resection margin clearance criteria with survival after surgery for cancer of esophagus. J Surg Oncol 2012;105(8):745–9.

30. Khan OA, Fitzgerald JJ, Soomro I, et al. Prognostic significance of circumferential resection margin involvement following oesophagectomy for cancer. Br J Cancer 2003;88(10):1549–52.

31. Suttie SA, Nanthakumaran S, Mofidi R, et al. The impact of operative approach for oesophageal cancer on outcome: the transhiatal approach may influence circumferential margin involvement. Eur J Surg Oncol 2012;38(2):157–65.

32. Williams VA, Peters JH. Adenocarcinoma of the gastroesophageal junction: benefits of an extended lymphadenectomy. Surg Oncol Clin N Am 2006; 15(4):765–80.

33. van Hagen P, Hulshof MC, van Lanschot JJ, et al. Preoperative chemoradiotherapy for esophageal or junctional cancer. N Engl J Med 2012;366:2074–84.

34. Kelsen DP, Ginsberg R, Pajak TF, et al. Chemotherapy followed by surgery compared with surgery alone for localized esophageal cancer. N Engl J Med 1998;339:1979–84.

35. Kim KT, Jeong O, Jung MR, et al. Outcomes of abdominal total gastrectomy for Type II and II

gastroesophageal junction tumors: single center's experience in Korea. J Gastric Cancer 2012;12(1): 36–42.

36. Papachristou DN, Agnanti N, D'Agostino H, et al. Histologically positive esophageal margin in the surgical treatment of gastric cancer. Am J Surg 1980; 139(5):711–3.

37. Johansson J, Djerf P, Oberg S, et al. Two different surgical approaches in the treatment of adenocarcinoma at the gastroesophageal junction. World J Surg 2008;32(6):1013–20.

38. Avella D, Garcia L, Hartman B, et al. Esophageal extension encountered during transhiatal resection of gastric or gastroesophageal tumors: attaining a negative margin. J Gastrointest Surg 2009;13(2): 368–73.

39. Mattioli S, Di Simone MP, Ferruzzi L, et al. Surgical therapy for adenocarcinoma of the cardia: modalities of recurrence and extension of resection. Dis Esophagus 2001;14(2):104–9.

40. Ito H, Clancy TE, Osteen RT, et al. Adenocarcinoma of the gastric cardia: what is the optimal surgical approach? J Am Coll Surg 2004;199(6):880–6.

41. Lam KY, Ma LT, Wong J. Measurement of extent of spread of oesophageal squamous carcinoma by serial sectioning. J Clin Pathol 1996;49(2):124–9.

42. Tsutsui S, Kuwano H, Watanabe M, et al. Resection margin for squamous cell carcinoma of the esophagus. Ann Surg 1995;222(2):193–202.

43. Kim SH, Karpeh MS, Klimstra DS, et al. Effect of microscopic resection line disease on gastric cancer survival. J Gastrointest Surg 1999;3:24–33.

Induction Therapy for Esophageal Cancer

Subroto Paul, MD, Nasser Altorki, MD*

KEYWORDS

- Esophageal cancer • Neoadjuvant therapy • Chemotherapy • Radiotherapy • Surgery

KEY POINTS

- Despite advances in treatment, long-term outcomes for esophageal cancer remain poor, with overall survival rates of between 15% and 35%.
- The objective of induction therapy is to improve overall and disease-free survival by enhancing locoregional disease control, as well as treating micrometastatic disease in the hope of preventing future systemic disease.
- Both induction chemotherapy and chemoradiation provide a modest survival advantage in comparison with surgical resection alone.
- Although meta-analyses suggest a small survival advantage to induction chemoradiation, there is no level-1 evidence to date supporting the superiority of induction chemoradiation over chemotherapy as the preferred neoadjuvant strategy.
- As the molecular biology of esophageal cancer is further elucidated, newer molecular targeted therapies will be developed, and may play a larger role in future trials.

INTRODUCTION

Despite advances in treatment, long-term outcomes for esophageal cancer remain poor, with overall survival rates of between 15% and 35%.[1–4] Poor long-term survival reflects locoregionally advanced disease (T1–2/N1–3 or T3–4/N0–3) or metastatic disease at presentation. Among patients undergoing surgical resection, 40% to 50% have stage III (T3N1–3, T4N0–3) disease.[1–4] Surgery alone results in poor locoregional control and poor long-term outcomes, with survival rates ranging from 10% to 30%. Induction therapy combining surgery with chemotherapy with or without radiotherapy attempts to improve long-term survival in these patients. This article examines the merits of various modalities of induction therapy for patients with locally advanced esophageal cancer.

RATIONALE FOR INDUCTION THERAPY

The objective of induction therapy is to improve overall and disease-free survival by enhancing locoregional disease control, as well as treating micrometastatic disease in the hope of preventing future systemic disease. Furthermore, induction therapy provides an in vivo assay to assess the biological behavior of the tumor. Patients with a significant response to induction therapy often have improved survival. Three major induction modalities have been used: preoperative radiotherapy, chemotherapy, or a combination of the two.

PREOPERATIVE RADIOTHERAPY FOLLOWED BY SURGERY

Six randomized controlled trials have been performed comparing preoperative radiotherapy

Disclosures: The authors have nothing to disclose.
Division of Thoracic Surgery, Department of Cardiothoracic Surgery, New York Presbyterian Hospital, Weill Cornell Medical College, New York, NY 10065, USA
* Corresponding author.
E-mail address: nkaltork@med.cornell.edu

followed by surgery with surgery alone.[5–9] The radiation dose varied in each of the trials (20–53 Gy) as did the interval between the cessation of therapy and surgical resection (1–6 weeks).[5–9] None of these trials demonstrated any benefit to preoperative radiotherapy. The Esophageal Cancer Collaborative Group reported a meta-analysis of 5 of these trials using aggregate data from a total of 1147 patients with a median follow-up of 9 years. Their results suggested a small absolute improvement in survival of 4% at 5 years.[10] A second meta-analysis conducted by Malthaner and colleagues[10–13] using 1-year survival data from all of these trials found no benefit from preoperative radiotherapy in comparison with surgery alone, with a hazard ratio (HR) of 1.01 (95% confidence interval [CI] 0.88–1.16). Given the results of the randomized trials and the conflicting results of the meta-analyses, there is no significant evidence supporting the role of induction radiotherapy for esophageal cancer.

INDUCTION CHEMOTHERAPY FOLLOWED BY SURGERY

Since 1980 at least 10 randomized trials have been conducted comparing induction chemotherapy with surgery alone.[14–20] This review focuses on the larger and most mature of these trials (**Table 1**).[18–20] In the intergroup trial (INT-113),

Kelsen and colleagues[19] compared the outcomes of 440 patients with stage I to III esophageal carcinoma (adenocarcinoma and squamous cell carcinoma) randomized to either 3 cycles of cisplatin and 5-fluorouracil (5-FU) followed by surgery (213 patients) or surgery alone (227 patients). Patients randomized to induction chemotherapy followed by surgery received additional postoperative chemotherapy (2 cycles of cisplatin/5-FU). In this trial, the complete pathologic response rate (pCR) was 2.5%, and there was no significant difference in either median or 2 year survival between the two arms of the study (14.9 months and 35% [chemotherapy + surgery] versus 16.1 months and 37% [surgery]; P = .53).[19] Long-term follow-up of this trial confirmed that there were no differences between treatment arms. However, the investigators found that long-term results showed that patients who had objective tumor regression after preoperative chemotherapy had improved survival.[21]

The European Medical Research Council (MRC OEO-2) trial randomized 802 patients with resectable esophageal cancer (either squamous cell carcinoma or adenocarcinoma) to 2 cycles of cisplatin and 5-FU followed by surgical resection or surgery alone.[18] In this trial, patients undergoing preoperative chemotherapy had higher rates of R0 resection than those who underwent surgery alone (60% [n = 233] vs 54% [n = 215]; P<.0001). When

Table 1
Trials of induction chemotherapy versus surgery

Authors,[Ref.] Year	No. of Patients	Chemotherapy	pCR (%)	Median Survival (mo)	5-Year Survival (%)	P Value
Roth et al,[14] 1988	C + S 19 S 20	Neo: Cis, Vin, Bleo Adj: Cis, Vin	NA	9 9	NA NA	NS
Nygaard et al,[15] 1992	C + S 50 S 41	Cis, Bleo	NA	8 8	3 (3 y) 9	NS
Schlag,[17] 1992	C + S 22 S 24	Cis, 5-FU	NA	10 10	NA	NS
Kelsen et al,[19] 1998	C + S 213 S 227	Cis, 5-FU Adj: Cis, 5-FU	2.5	14.9 16.1	35 (2 y) 37	NS
Ancona et al,[16] 2001	C + S 47 S 47	Cis,5-FU	13	25 24	34 22	NS
MRC,[18] 2002	C + S 400 S 402	Cis, 5-FU	4	16.8 13.3	43 (2 y) 34	.004
Cunningham et al,[20] 2006	C + S 250 S 253	Cis, 5-FU, Epi Adj: Cis, 5-FU, Epi	0	24 20	36.3 23.0	.009
Ychou et al,[24] 2011	C + S 113 S 111	Cis, 5-FU	NA	NA NA	38 24	.02

Abbreviations: Adj, adjuvant; Bleo, bleomycin; C, chemotherapy; Cis, cisplatin; Epi, epirubicin; 5-FU, 5-fluorouracil; MRC, Medical Research Council; NA, no data available; Neo, neoadjuvant; NS, not significant; pCR, complete pathologic response; S, surgery; Vin, vincristine.
Data from Refs.[14–20,24]

comparing the postresection pathologic specimens, these patients also had smaller tumors, less frequent invasion of surrounding tissue, and less lymph node involvement than patients who had surgery alone. Both median survival and 2-year overall survival were improved in patients enrolled in the induction chemotherapy arm (16.8 months vs 13.3 months [P<.004], 43% vs 34% [P<.004], respectively).[18] Long-term follow-up of this trial showed the survival benefit of preoperative chemotherapy and surgery compared with surgery alone (HR 0.84, 95% CI: 0.72–0.98; P = .03) to be maintained. The treatment benefit was evident for both adenocarcinoma and squamous cell carcinoma of the esophagus.[22] The survival advantage seen in the MRC trial over the INT-113 trial may be due to the larger sample size in the European trial, which enables small differences in treatment outcomes to be detected, as well as the fact that more patients (92% vs 80%) proceeded to surgical resection in the MRC trial.[18,19]

The MRC Adjuvant Gastric Infusional Chemotherapy (MAGIC) trial randomized 503 patients with gastric cancer and adenocarcinoma of the esophagus and gastroesophageal junction, stage II or higher, to 3 cycles of epirubicin, cisplatin, and 5-FU followed by surgery, with an additional 3 cycles of chemotherapy postoperatively (n = 250) or surgery alone.[20] Most patients in this trial had gastric cancer, with only 26% of patients in both arms having carcinoma of the lower esophagus or gastroesophageal junction.[20] This trial, like the MRC trial, showed that patients undergoing preoperative chemotherapy had smaller tumors (medial maximal tumor diameter: 3 cm vs 5 cm; P<.001), less nodal involvement (for gastric cancer), and less advanced pathologic stage than those who underwent surgery alone. The MAGIC trial also showed, like the MRC trial, that induction chemotherapy led to a significant survival advantage, with an improvement in median survival (24 months vs 20 months; P<.009) and 5-year overall survival (36% vs 23%; P<.009).[20] Any benefit from chemotherapy is attributed to its use in the induction setting, because only 42% completed adjuvant chemotherapy. The major criticism of the results of the MAGIC trial is that the majority of patients in the trial have gastric cancer; and hence many argue that its results should not be extended to esophageal cancer. However, the multivariable analysis showed that the survival advantage conferred by induction chemotherapy was unchanged after adjustment for tumor site.

Further support for a survival benefit from neoadjuvant chemotherapy and surgery comes from the French Intergroup Trial (FFCD/FNLCC-94012). In this trial, Ychou and colleagues[23,24] randomized 224 patients with adenocarcinoma of the distal esophagus (n = 25), gastroesophageal junction (n = 144), and stomach (n = 55), stage II or greater, to 2 to 3 cycles of 5-FU and cisplatin followed by surgery with 1 to 4 additional cycles of the same chemotherapy postoperatively, or surgery alone. In contrast to the MAGIC trial, 75% of patients in this trial had adenocarcinoma of the distal esophagus and gastroesophageal junction. This trial also demonstrated a survival advantage to preoperative chemotherapy, with improved 5-year disease-free survival (34% vs 19%; P = .003) and overall survival (38% vs 24%; P = .02) in the treatment arm.[23,24] Treatment-related toxicity was similar in both groups.[23,24]

Additional clinical evidence for the use of induction chemotherapy comes from meta-analysis data. As multiple meta-analyses have been published since 2003, only the more comprehensive analyses are discussed here. Eleven randomized trials with a total of 2051 patients were analyzed in a Cochrane review in 2003.[11] In this analysis the cumulative response rate to chemotherapy was 36%, with 3% of patients having a pCR. No difference in overall survival was seen at 1 to 2 years. A survival advantage was detected at 3 years with statistical significance achieved at 5 years.[11] In 2007, Thirion and colleagues[25] presented pooled individual patient data from 9 randomized trials performed from the early 1980s to the mid-1990s. This analysis showed that preoperative chemotherapy was associated with a statistically significant improvement in disease-free and overall survival (4.3% and 4.1%, respectively). In a recent meta-analysis published in 2011, Sjoquist and colleagues[3] updated their previous work to include studies published since 2006.[4] In their updated analysis, which included randomized controlled trials from 1982 onward, a modest but significant improvement in absolute 2-year survival of 5.1% (HR 0.79–0.96; P = .005) was found with induction chemotherapy in comparison with surgery alone. However, the survival benefit from induction chemotherapy seems to be dependent on histology, with the strongest benefit found in those with adenocarcinoma of the esophagus. Their analysis excluded data from the MAGIC trial, as most patients in this trial underwent gastrectomy. The investigators comment that the survival advantage from induction chemotherapy remains even when the results of the MAGIC esophageal carcinoma subgroup were included in their analysis.[3,4]

Based on the results of at least 3 well-powered randomized trials and the meta-analyses by Thirion and colleagues[25] and Sjoquist and colleagues,[3] there appears to be sufficient evidence to suggest a modest benefit from induction chemotherapy in the treatment of locally advanced esophageal carcinoma over surgery alone; especially for those with adenocarcinoma of the esophagus.

INDUCTION CHEMORADIATION FOLLOWED BY SURGERY

The addition of radiotherapy to induction chemotherapy regimens adds another modality for locoregional control. By increasing the rate of pCR, preoperative chemoradiation could theoretically reduce local recurrence rates and improve survival. There have been numerous nonrandomized and randomized trials evaluating induction chemoradiation. Most of these trials used chemotherapy based on cisplatin and 5-FU, with radiotherapy doses varying from 20 to 40 Gy.

Interpreting the results of these trials is difficult because of their small sample sizes, the variability of preoperative chemoradiation regimens, and the incomplete and often variable preoperative staging modalities used. These trials also encompass a wider time frame, with some trials completed in the early 1980s and 1990s. Clearly there have been significant improvements in surgical technique, chemotherapeutic agents, radiotherapy protocols, and preoperative staging modalities since this time. Nevertheless, examination of the sentinel trials and their pooled analysis provide some insight into the efficacy of neoadjuvant chemoradiation in the treatment of esophageal cancer.

At least 12 major randomized trials evaluating neoadjuvant chemoradiation took place in the period 1992 to 2011,[15,26–36] and these are listed in **Table 2**. Walsh and colleagues[28] randomized 113 patients with esophageal adenocarcinoma to surgery alone or 2 cycles of cisplatin/5-FU and 40 Gy of radiotherapy followed by surgical resection. After preoperative chemoradiation, more patients had either a pCR (25%) or node-negative disease (58% vs 16%). Three-year survival was significantly improved in the multimodality arm

Table 2
Trials of induction chemoradiotherapy versus surgery

Authors,[Ref.] Year	No. of Patients	CRT	pCR (%)	Median Survival (mo)	3-Year Survival (%)	P Value
Nygaard et al,[15] 1992	S 41 CRT + S 47	Cis + Bleo 35 Gy	NA	7.5 7.5	9 17	NS
Le Prise et al,[26] 1994	S 45 CRT + S 41	Cis + 5-FU 20 Gy	10	10 10	14 19	NS
Apinop et al,[27] 1994	S 34 CRT +S 35	Cis + 5-FU 40 Gy	NA	7 10	20 26	NS
Walsh et al,[28] 1996	S 55 CRT + S 58	Cis + 5-FU 40 Gy	25	11 16	6 32	.01
Bosset et al,[30] 1997	S 139 CRT + S 143	Cis 37 Gy	26	19 19	37 39	NS
Law et al,[29] 1998	S 30 CRT + S 30	Cis + 5-FU 40 Gy	25	27 26	NA NA	NS
Urba et al,[31] 2001	S 50 CRT + S 50	Cis + 5-Fu + Vin 45 Gy	28	18 17	16 30	NS
Burmeister et al,[33] 2005	S 128 CRT + S 128	Cis + 5-FU 35 Gy	16	22 19	NA NA	NS
Tepper et al,[33] 2005	S 26 CRT + S 30	Cis + 5-FU 50.4 Gy	40	22 54	16 39	<.008
Lv et al,[34] 2010	S 80 CRT + S 80	Carbo + paclitaxel 40 Gy	NA	NA NA	51.3 63.5	.0389
Mariette et al,[36] 2010	S 98 CRT + S 97	Cis + 5-FU 45 Gy	32.6	43.8 31.8	NA NA	.66
van der Gaast et al,[35] 2011	S 188 CRT + S 175	Carbo + paclitaxel 41.4 Gy	32.6	26 49	48 59	.011

Abbreviations: Bleo, bleomycin; Carbo, carboplatin; Cis, cisplatin; CRT, chemoradiotherapy; 5-FU, 5-fluorouracil; NA, no data available; NS, not significant; pCR, complete pathologic response; S, surgery; Vin, vincristine.
Data from Refs.[15,26–36]

in comparison with surgery alone (32% vs 6%; P<.01). There have been several criticisms of this trial, primarily directed at inadequate preoperative staging and unusually poor survival in the surgery-alone arm (6% at 3 years). As most surgical series demonstrate a 3-year survival of at least 20% with surgery alone, this suggests a potential imbalance between the two arms of the trial favoring the tri-modality arm.[37–40] Despite these limitations, until 2006 this study was the only randomized trial demonstrating a survival benefit from preoperative chemoradiation.[28,37–41]

Randomized studies performed by Urba and colleagues, Nygaard and colleagues, Le Prise and colleagues, Burmeister and colleagues, Bosset and colleagues, and Aninop and colleagues[15,26,27,30,31,33] were unable to demonstrate a statistically significant survival benefit from induction chemoradiation (**Table 2**). These trials instead suggested a potential benefit from preoperative chemoradiation based on secondary end point or post hoc subgroup analysis.

Bosset and colleagues[30] randomized 282 patients with squamous cell carcinoma, stage I and II, to surgery alone or cisplatin and 37 Gy followed by surgery. A pCR was seen in 26% patients receiving the treatment arm. There was an improvement in 3-year disease-free, but not overall, survival in patients receiving neoadjuvant chemoradiation (40% vs 28%; P = .003). In this trial, induction chemoradiation was associated with a higher postoperative mortality than was surgery alone (12.3% vs 3.6%; P = .012).

Burmeister and colleagues[33] randomized 256 patients with esophageal carcinoma to either neo-adjuvant cisplatin and 5-FU and concurrent 35 Gy of radiotherapy followed by surgery, or surgery alone. Sixty percent of patients had adenocarcinoma, stage I to III, as determined by endoscopy and computed tomography. The pCR was 16%, with higher rates of pCR in patients with squamous cell carcinoma than with adenocarcinoma (27% vs 9%; P = .02). In this study, neither survival nor disease-free survival was statistically different between the two treatment arms. Post hoc subgroup analysis demonstrated that neoadjuvant chemoradiation improved disease-free survival in patients with squamous cell carcinoma (HR 0.47, 95% CI 0.25–0.86; P = .014), with a trend toward improved recurrence-free survival for those with adenocarcinoma.

Single-agent or a single cycle of chemotherapy was given in the Bosset and Burmeister trials.[30,33,37–41] In the Bosset trial, cisplatin was administered as single dose before radiation in 2 1-week courses, whereas in the Burmeister study a single cycle of cisplatin and 5-FU was given.

The lack of any observed survival benefit in these 2 trials may be due to these suboptimal chemotherapy regimens administered in each trial.

The American Cancer and Acute Leukemia Group B (CALGB)-9781 trial evaluating chemoradiation was closed prematurely owing to poor accrual, with only 56 patients enrolled before closure. The planned accrual was 500 patients. The majority of patients (75%) had esophageal adenocarcinoma stage I to III. Patients in this study were randomized to 2 cycles of chemotherapy with 5-FU and 50.4 Gy of radiation before surgery, or surgery alone.[32,37] Despite the small sample size, this trial demonstrated that induction chemoradiation was associated with an improvement in both median survival (4.5 years vs 1.8 years; P = .02) and 5-year overall survival (39% vs 16%; P<.008) in the treatment arm.[32,37] The results of this trial are difficult to validate, given its small sample size and its poor accrual leading to premature closure.

Van der Gaast and colleagues[35,42] enrolled 368 patients with resectable T2-3N0-1 esophageal cancer (75% adenocarcinoma) to 5 weeks of carboplatin and paclitaxel and concurrent 41.4-Gy radiotherapy followed by resection, or resection alone.[35,42] Follow-up data were obtained for 366 patients. There was a pCR of 29%, with an improvement in median survival (49.4 vs 24.0 months, P = .011). Overall survival was significantly better in the patients undergoing surgical resection after chemoradiotherapy (HR 0.657, 95% CI 0.495–0.871; P = .003). Subgroup analysis by histology demonstrated an increased survival benefit for the patients with squamous carcinoma (adjusted HR 0.422, 95% CI 0.226–0.788; P = .007) but only a marginal benefit for adenocarcinoma patients (adjusted HR 0.741, 95% CI 0.536–1.024; P = .07) who underwent chemoradiation followed by surgery. Treatment-related toxicity was limited in this trial, with in-hospital mortality of 4% in both arms of the trial.[35,42] The investigators suggest that their results provide compelling evidence that induction chemoradiation should be the standard of care for locally advanced esophageal cancer, particularly for squamous cell carcinoma.

Multiple meta-analyses evaluating induction chemoradiotherapy have been reported, including those by Fiorica and colleagues, Urschel and Vasan, Greer and colleagues, Malthaner and colleagues, and, more recently, Sjoquist and colleagues.[12,43–45] Each of these studies reported a small survival benefit from preoperative chemoradiation.[12,43–45]

Fiorica and colleagues[44] pooled patients from 6 randomized controlled trials comparing induction chemoradiation and surgery with surgery alone (those by the groups of Nygaard, Le Prise, Apinop, Walsh, Bosset, and Urba)[15,26–28,30,31] encompassing 764 patients. Trials included patients with only resectable esophageal carcinoma. Only 1 of the 6 studies included in the meta-analysis (Walsh and colleagues[28]) showed a statistically significant survival benefit after induction chemoradiation. This analysis demonstrated 3-year mortality to be lower after chemoradiation and surgery compared with surgery alone (odds ratio [OR] 0.53, 95% CI 0.31–0.92; $P = .025$). However, postoperative mortality was doubled after chemoradiation and surgery (OR 2.10; 95% CI 1.18–3.73; $P = .01$).[44] Greer and colleagues[45] pooled the same trials and reached similar conclusions. As both of these studies did not analyze individual patient data but rather group averages, any small therapeutic benefit from chemoradiation may have been lost in the statistical analysis.

Urschel and Vasan[45] combined data from the 6 trials analyzed by Fiorica and colleagues and Greer and colleagues, as well as 3 additional trials.[29,33,46] These trials included the results of 1116 patients and were graded for quality using the 5-point Jadad scale.[43] No benefit was found with the addition of induction chemoradiation to surgery until 3 years were reached (OR 0.66, 95% CI 0.47–0.92; $P = .016$). A trend toward increased postoperative mortality with induction chemoradiation was seen (OR 1.63, 95% CI 0.99–2.68; $P = .053$). In another meta-analysis by Malthaner and colleagues,[12] 3-year mortality was lower for patients receiving induction chemoradiation (OR 0.87, 95% CI 0.80–0.96; $P = .004$). Although individual patient data was obtained to some extent in both of these meta-analyses, this was not possible for most of the trials analyzed. Most of the results in both of these studies are based on summary estimates, which seriously limit the strength of the conclusions reached by Urschel and Vasan[45] and Malthaner and colleagues[12]

In 2011, Sjoquist and colleagues[3] updated their meta-analysis from 2007 to now include 13 randomized trials of induction chemoradiotherapy and surgery versus surgery alone. The investigators used the HR from each trial or from individual patient data to calculate 2-year survival estimates for each treatment arm. Neoadjuvant chemoradiation led to an absolute survival benefit at 2 years of 8.7% with a pooled HR of 0.78 ($P<.0001$).[3] The survival benefits of chemoradiation were seen in patients with both squamous cell carcinoma and adenocarcinoma. The meta-analysis did not find evidence to support that the benefits of induction chemoradiation were offset by surgical or in-hospital 30-day mortality.[3]

INDUCTION CHEMOTHERAPY FOLLOWED BY SURGERY VERSUS INDUCTION CHEMORADIATION FOLLOWED BY SURGERY

Meta-analysis data suggest that induction chemoradiation may confer a small survival advantage over induction chemotherapy for locoregionally advanced esophageal cancer. Randomized trials comparing the 2 regimens directly are limited. Hence, the question remains as to which regimen constitutes the optimal preoperative therapy. The Preoperative Chemotherapy or Radiochemotherapy in Esophagogastric Adenocarcinoma Trial (POET) trial conducted by the German Esophageal Cancer Study Group attempts to directly answer this question.[47] In this trial, patients with stage T3-4NxM0 adenocarcinoma of the esophagus were randomized to either induction chemotherapy only, with 2.5 cycles of cisplatin and 5-FU, or 2 courses of cisplatin and 5-FU followed by 3 weeks of chemoradiotherapy (30 Gy, cisplatin, and etoposide).[47] Esophagectomy was planned 3 to 4 weeks after the end of preoperative therapy in each arm. The study was closed early owing to poor accrual with a total of 120 eligible patients randomly assigned, of whom 90 patients underwent surgical resection. A pCR was found in 2.5% of patients who received neoadjuvant chemotherapy in comparison with 17% of patients who received neoadjuvant chemoradiation ($P = .06$).[47] However, this increase in pCR did not translate into a survival benefit (median survival 32.8 vs 21.1 months, 3-year survival 43% vs 27%; $P = .14$ for chemoradiation vs chemotherapy). Although this study was underpowered, these results suggest that induction chemoradiation may be marginally superior to induction chemotherapy in treating locally advanced esophageal cancer. This small survival benefit, however, may come at the cost of an increased postoperative mortality (8.3% vs 3.3% for preoperative chemoradiation and chemotherapy, respectively).

In another trial presented by Burmeister and colleagues, 65 patients were randomized to receive either induction chemotherapy with cisplatin and 5-FU, or induction chemoradiation with the same agents and 35 Gy of radiation followed by surgical resection.[48] Although the pCR was higher in the chemoradiation arm (31% vs 8%; $P = .01$), there was no difference in overall survival.[48] The study was underpowered to demonstrate small differences between the treatment arms.

FUTURE DIRECTIONS: INCORPORATING TARGETED THERAPIES

Despite the current modalities of induction therapy, patients often relapse with distant metastatic disease. In an effort to provide more effective treatment, the inclusion of specific molecular targeted therapies into induction regimens is currently being evaluated. Anti–epidermal growth factor receptor (EGFR) antibodies have received considerable interest as potential agents. Evidence from phase III trials in head and neck cancer in which cetuximab (anti-EGFR antibody) was used suggest that concurrently targeting EGFR may increase the efficacy of chemoradiation regimens.[49] The addition of cetuximab to radiation therapy nearly doubled median survival time from 28 to 54 months in this trial.[49] The Swiss Group for Clinical Cancer Research (SAKK) conducted a phase II trial investigating the toxicity of cetuximab as part of chemoradiotherapy regimen for esophageal cancer. Patients received 2 3-week cycles of cisplatin, docetaxel, and cetuximab followed by 45 Gy radiotherapy and concurrent cisplatin and cetuximab.[50] Twenty-eight patients (15 adenocarcinoma and 13 squamous cell carcinoma) were enrolled, with 24 completing the entire regimen. No limiting toxicity was seen during therapy. However, grade 3 toxicity occurred in 54% (n = 15) and consisted of esophagitis (n = 7), anorexia (n = 3), fatigue (n = 3), and thrombosis (n = 2). An R0 surgical resection was performed in 25 patients. Postoperative complications included infections (n = 10; 40%), anastomotic leaks (n = 3; 12%), and pulmonary embolism (n = 2; 8%). Sixty-eight percent (n = 19) showed complete or near complete pathologic regression. There were no 30-day deaths or treatment-related deaths in 12 months.[50] This trial showed the feasibility of adding anti-EGFR treatment to induction modalities for esophageal cancer, although with some grade 3 toxicity. However, the efficacy of this treatment is yet to be determined.

ACOSOG-Z405, another phase II trial, presented only in abstract form, examined the role of panitumumab, another anti-EGFR agent. This trial enrolled patients to receive cisplatin, docetaxel, and panitumumab for 2 weeks followed by cisplatin, docetaxel, panitumumab, and 5040 cGy radiotherapy for 3 weeks with subsequent surgery.[51] The trial's primary end point was pCR, a surrogate for improved survival. Of the 65 eligible patients, 58 underwent surgery. Of these patients, the pCR rate was 32.8%. Twenty-three percent of patients (n = 16) had a grade 4 adverse events that were treatment related. Although this trial also showed the feasibility of adding anti-EGFR therapy, the high rate of grade 4 adverse events is disappointing.[51] Long-term results have not been reported.

Similar conclusions have been reached in other phase II trials examining the addition of either cetuximab or panitumumab to chemoradiation regimens.[52,53] As the molecular biology of esophageal cancer is further elucidated, newer molecular targeted therapies will be developed and may play a larger role in future trials.

SUMMARY

Long-term outcomes for esophageal cancer remain poor, with the vast majority of patients presenting with locoregionally advanced disease. Surgery alone provides inadequate locoregional control and fails to address micrometastatic disease that is potentially present before resection. Both induction chemotherapy and chemoradiation provide a modest but clear survival advantage compared with surgical resection alone. Although meta-analyses suggest a small survival advantage over induction chemoradiation, there remains no level-1 evidence to date supporting the superiority of induction chemoradiation over chemotherapy as the preferred neoadjuvant strategy. Collectively, these results demonstrate that improvements in survival with induction strategies are modest: 8.7% improvement in 2-year survival at best. Improved chemotherapeutic and radiotherapy regimens are clearly needed.

REFERENCES

1. Devesa SS, Blot WJ, Fraumeni JF Jr. Changing patterns in the incidence of esophageal and gastric carcinoma in the United States. Cancer 1998; 83(10):2049–53.

2. Enzinger PC, Mayer RJ. Esophageal cancer. N Engl J Med 2003;349(23):2241–52.

3. Sjoquist KM, Burmeister BH, Smithers BM, et al. Survival after neoadjuvant chemotherapy or chemoradiotherapy for resectable oesophageal carcinoma: an updated meta-analysis. Lancet Oncol 2011;12(7):681–92.

4. Gebski V, Burmeister B, Smithers BM, et al. Survival benefits from neoadjuvant chemoradiotherapy or chemotherapy in oesophageal carcinoma: a meta-analysis. Lancet Oncol 2007;8(3):226–34.

5. Launois B, Delarue D, Campion JP, et al. Preoperative radiotherapy for carcinoma of the esophagus. Surg Gynecol Obstet 1981;153(5):690–2.

6. Gignoux M, Roussel A, Paillot B, et al. The value of preoperative radiotherapy in esophageal cancer: results of a study by the EORTC. Recent Results Cancer Res 1988;110:1–13.

7. Wang M, Gu XZ, Yin WB, et al. Randomized clinical trial on the combination of preoperative irradiation and surgery in the treatment of esophageal carcinoma: report on 206 patients. Int J Radiat Oncol Biol Phys 1989;16(2):325–7.

8. Arnott SJ, Duncan W, Kerr GR, et al. Low dose preoperative radiotherapy for carcinoma of the oesophagus: results of a randomized clinical trial. Radiother Oncol 1992;24(2):108–13.

9. Fok M, McShane J, Law S, et al. Prospective randomised study in the treatment of oesophageal carcinoma. Asian J Surg 1994;17:223–9.

10. Arnott SJ, Duncan W, Gignoux M, et al. Preoperative radiotherapy in esophageal carcinoma: a meta-analysis using individual patient data (Oesophageal Cancer Collaborative Group). Int J Radiat Oncol Biol Phys 1998;41(3):579–83.

11. Malthaner R, Fenlon D. Preoperative chemotherapy for resectable thoracic esophageal cancer. Cochrane Database Syst Rev 2003;(4):CD001556.

12. Malthaner RA, Wong RK, Rumble RB, et al. Neoadjuvant or adjuvant therapy for resectable esophageal cancer: a systematic review and meta-analysis. BMC Med 2004;2(1):35.

13. Arnott SJ, Duncan W, Gignoux M, et al. Preoperative radiotherapy for esophageal carcinoma. Cochrane Database Syst Rev 2005;(4):CD001799.

14. Roth JA, Pass HI, Flanagan MM, et al. Randomized clinical trial of preoperative and postoperative adjuvant chemotherapy with cisplatin, vindesine, and bleomycin for carcinoma of the esophagus. J Thorac Cardiovasc Surg 1988;96(2):242–8.

15. Nygaard K, Hagen S, Hansen HS, et al. Pre-operative radiotherapy prolongs survival in operable esophageal carcinoma: a randomized, multicenter study of pre-operative radiotherapy and chemotherapy. The second Scandinavian trial in esophageal cancer. World J Surg 1992;16(6):1104–9 [discussion: 1110].

16. Ancona E, Ruol A, Santi S, et al. Only pathologic complete response to neoadjuvant chemotherapy improves significantly the long term survival of patients with resectable esophageal squamous cell carcinoma: final report of a randomized, controlled trial of preoperative chemotherapy versus surgery alone. Cancer 2001;91(11):2165–74.

17. Schlag PM. Randomized trial of preoperative chemotherapy for squamous cell cancer of the esophagus. The Chirurgische Arbeitsgemeinschaft Fuer Onkologie der Deutschen Gesellschaft Fuer Chirurgie Study Group. Arch Surg 1992;127(12):1446–50.

18. Medical Research Council Oesophageal Cancer Working Group. Surgical resection with or without preoperative chemotherapy in oesophageal cancer: a randomised controlled trial. Lancet 2002;359(9319):1727–33.

19. Kelsen DP, Ginsberg R, Pajak TF, et al. Chemotherapy followed by surgery compared with surgery alone for localized esophageal cancer. N Engl J Med 1998;339(27):1979–84.

20. Cunningham D, Allum WH, Stenning SP, et al. Perioperative chemotherapy versus surgery alone for resectable gastroesophageal cancer. N Engl J Med 2006;355(1):11–20.

21. Kelsen DP, Winter KA, Gunderson LL, et al. Long-term results of RTOG trial 8911 (USA Intergroup 113): a random assignment trial comparison of chemotherapy followed by surgery compared with surgery alone for esophageal cancer. J Clin Oncol 2007;25(24):3719–25.

22. Allum WH, Stenning SP, Bancewicz J, et al. Long-term results of a randomized trial of surgery with or without preoperative chemotherapy in esophageal cancer. J Clin Oncol 2009;27(30):5062–7.

23. Boige V, Pignon J, Saint-Aubert B, et al. Final results of a randomized trial comparing preoperative 5-fluorouracil (F)/cisplatin (P) to surgery alone in adenocarcinoma of stomach and lower esophagus (ASLE): FNLCC ACCORD07-FFCD 9703 trial. J Clin Oncol 2007;25(18S):4510.

24. Ychou M, Boige V, Pignon JP, et al. Perioperative chemotherapy compared with surgery alone for resectable gastroesophageal adenocarcinoma: an FNCLCC and FFCD multicenter phase III trial. J Clin Oncol 2011;29(13):1715–21.

25. Thirion PG, Michiels S, Le Maitre A, et al. Individual patient data-based meta-analysis assessing preoperative chemotherapy in resectable oesophageal adenocarcinoma. J Clin Oncol 2007;25(18S):4512.

26. Le Prise E, Etienne PL, Meunier B, et al. A randomized study of chemotherapy, radiation therapy, and surgery versus surgery for localized squamous cell carcinoma of the esophagus. Cancer 1994;73(7):1779–84.

27. Apinop C, Puttisak P, Preecha N. A prospective study of combined therapy in esophageal cancer. Hepatogastroenterology 1994;41(4):391–3.

28. Walsh TN, Noonan N, Hollywood D, et al. A comparison of multimodal therapy and surgery for esophageal adenocarcinoma. N Engl J Med 1996;335(7):462–7.

29. Law S, Kwong DL, Tung HM. Preoperative chemoradiation for squamous cell esophageal cancer: a prospective randomized trial (abstract). Can J Gastroenterol 1998;12(Suppl B):161.

30. Bosset JF, Gignoux M, Triboulet JP, et al. Chemoradiotherapy followed by surgery compared with surgery alone in squamous-cell cancer of the esophagus. N Engl J Med 1997;337(3):161–7.

31. Urba SG, Orringer MB, Turrisi A, et al. Randomized trial of preoperative chemoradiation versus surgery alone in patients with locoregional esophageal carcinoma. J Clin Oncol 2001;19(2):305–13.

32. Tepper J, Krasna MJ, Niedzwicki D. Superiority of trimodality therapy to surgery alone in esophageal cancer: results of CALGB 9781. J Clin Oncol 2006;24:181.

33. Burmeister BH, Smithers BM, Gebski V, et al. Surgery alone versus chemoradiotherapy followed by surgery for resectable cancer of the oesophagus: a randomised controlled phase III trial. Lancet Oncol 2005;6(9):659–68.

34. Lv J, Cao XF, Zhu B, et al. Long-term efficacy of perioperative chemoradiotherapy on esophageal squamous cell carcinoma. World J Gastroenterol 2010;16(13):1649–54.

35. van der Gaast A, van Hagen P, Hulshof M, et al. Effect of preoperative concurrent radiotherapy on survival of patients with resectable esophageal or esophagogastric junction cancer: results from a multicenter randomized phase III study. J Clin Oncol 2011;28(Suppl 15) [abstract 4004].

36. Mariette C, Seitz JF, Maillard B, et al. Surgery alone versus chemoradiotherapy followed by surgery for localized esophageal cancer; analysis of a randomized controlled phase III trial FFCD 9901. Proc Am Soc Clin Oncol 2010;28(Suppl 15) [abstract 4005].

37. Ilson DH. Cancer of the gastroesophageal junction: combined modality therapy. Surg Oncol Clin N Am 2006;15(4):803–24.

38. Yoon HH, Gibson MK. Combined-modality therapy for esophageal and gastroesophageal junction cancers. Curr Oncol Rep 2007;9(3):184–92.

39. Piraino A, Vita ML, Tessitore A, et al. Neoadjuvant therapy for esophageal cancer: surgical considerations. Rays 2006;31(1):37–45.

40. McKian KP, Miller RC, Cassivi SD, et al. Curing patients with locally advanced esophageal cancer: an update on multimodality therapy. Dis Esophagus 2006;19(6):448–53.

41. Shinoda M, Hatooka S, Mori S, et al. Clinical aspects of multimodality therapy for resectable locoregional esophageal cancer. Ann Thorac Cardiovasc Surg 2006;12(4):234–41.

42. van Hagen P, Hulshof MC, van Lanschot JJ, et al. Preoperative chemoradiotherapy for esophageal or junctional cancer. N Engl J Med 2012;366(22):2074–84.

43. Urschel JD, Vasan H. A meta-analysis of randomized controlled trials that compared neoadjuvant chemoradiation and surgery to surgery alone for resectable esophageal cancer. Am J Surg 2003;185(6):538–43.

44. Fiorica F, Di Bona D, Schepis F, et al. Preoperative chemoradiotherapy for oesophageal cancer: a systematic review and meta-analysis. Gut 2004;53(7):925–30.

45. Greer SE, Goodney PP, Sutton JE, et al. Neoadjuvant chemoradiotherapy for esophageal carcinoma: a meta-analysis. Surgery 2005;137(2):172–7.

46. Walsh TN, McDonnell CO, Mulligan ED. Multimodal therapy versus surgery alone for squamous cell carcinoma of esophagus. Gastroenterology 2000;118(Suppl 2):A1008.

47. Stahl M, Walz MK, Stuschke M, et al. Preoperative chemotherapy (CTX) versus preoperative chemoradiotherapy (CRTZ) in locally advanced esophagogastric adenocarcinomas: first results of a randomized phase III trial. J Clin Oncol 2007;25(18S):4511.

48. Burmeister BH, Thomas JM, Burmeister EA, et al. Is concurrent radiation therapy required in patients receiving preoperative chemotherapy for adenocarcinoma of the oesophagus? A randomised phase II trial. Eur J Cancer 2011;47(3):354–60.

49. Bonner JA, Harari PM, Giralt J, et al. Radiotherapy plus cetuximab for squamous-cell carcinoma of the head and neck. N Engl J Med 2006;354:567–78.

50. Ruhstaller T, Pless M, Dietrich D, et al. Cetuximab in combination with chemoradiotherapy before surgery in patients with resectable, locally advanced esophageal carcinoma: a prospective, multicenter phase IB/II Trial (SAKK 75/06). J Clin Oncol 2011;29(6):626–31.

51. Reed C, Decker P, Schefter T, et al. A phase II study of neoadjuvant therapy with cisplatin, docetaxel, panitumumab plus radiation therapy followed by surgery in patients with locally advanced adenocarcinoma of the distal esophagus (ACOSOG Z4051). J Clin Oncol 2012;30(Suppl) [abstract 4062].

52. De Vita F, Orditura M, Martinelli E, et al. A multicenter phase II study of induction chemotherapy with FOLFOX-4 and cetuximab followed by radiation and cetuximab in locally advanced oesophageal cancer. Br J Cancer 2011;104(3):427–32.

53. Kordes S, Richel D, van Berge Henegouwen MI, et al. Multicenter phase II study combining panitumumab with chemoradiation followed by surgery for patients with operable esophageal cancer (PACT-study). J Clin Oncol 2012;30(Suppl) [abstract 4094].

Neoadjuvant Chemotherapy or Chemoradiotherapy for Locally Advanced Esophageal Cancer

B. Mark Smithers, MBBS, FRACS, FRCSEng, FRCSEd*,
Iain Thomson, MBBS, FRACS

KEYWORDS

- Esophageal cancer • Esophagogastric junction adenocarcinoma • Neoadjuvant chemotherapy
- Neoadjuvant chemoradiation • Pathologic complete response • Esophagectomy

KEY POINTS

- Neoadjuvant therapy with chemotherapy (CT) or chemoradiotherapy (CRT) improves survival in patients with locally advanced esophageal cancer.
- There is no robust study that has directly compared neoadjuvant CT with neoadjuvant CRT for patients with squamous cell carcinoma or adenocarcinoma.
- Treatment decisions should be based on histology and local staging using endoscopic ultrasonography, along with local and systemic staging with computed tomography/fluorodeoxyglucose positron emission tomography.
- The decision relating to the ability to resect may include considerations such as the association of the primary cancer with major anatomic structures.
- The future will involve the assessment of newer chemotherapeutic agents, which have a greater effect on occult disease.

OVERVIEW

The improvement in patient outcomes from esophageal cancer is a result of better cancer staging and patient selection for surgery along with the concentration of patient care into specialist centers and improvement in perioperative management. In parallel with positive changes in general management, cancer outcomes have improved after phase II and III trials exploring the role of chemotherapy (CT) and radiotherapy, in association with surgery for this disease.

Adjuvant therapy
- No clear evidence for single-modality, postoperative adjuvant therapy for esophageal cancer.

- Single trial reports benefit for postoperative chemoradiotherapy (CRT) in patients with squamous cell carcinoma (SCC).[1]

Neoadjuvant therapy
- No clear role for preoperative radiotherapy alone followed by resection[2]
- Survival benefit in trials assessing neoadjuvant CT (pre-CT)[3–7]
- Survival benefit in trials assessing neoadjuvant CRT (pre-CRT)[1,8–10]
- Treatment-related mortality occurs associated with pre-CT(1.7%) and pre-CRT(3.4%)[11]

Recent meta-analysis[12]: 21 randomized controlled trials (RCTs)/4188 patients: 9 pre-CT versus surgery alone[3,5,6,13–19]; 12

Disclosures: The authors have nothing to disclose.
Upper GI, Soft Tissue Unit, Discipline of Surgery, Princess Alexandra Hospital, The University of Queensland, Ipswich Road, Buranda, Brisbane 4102, Australia
* Corresponding author.
E-mail address: m.smithers@uq.edu.au

pre-CRT versus surgery alone[1,4,8–10,20–26] and 2 pre-CT versus pre-CRT.[27,28]

- Pre-CRT: whole-group hazard ratio 0.78 (P = .0001). Adenocarcinoma (AC), 0.75 (P = .02); SCC, 0.8 (P = .02).
- Pre-CT: whole-group hazard ratio 0.87 (P = .005). AC, 0.83 (P = .01); SCC, 0.92 (P = .18).
- Comparing the treatment arms of all trials: no difference in overall survival between pre-CRT or pre-CT.

The trials assessed in the most recent meta-analysis included patients with SCC, AC, AC of the esophagogastric junction (EGJAC) and had different CT regimens and different radiation doses and methods of delivery, along with the earlier trials using variable staging and with poor outcomes in the control arm of surgery alone. This variability and heterogeneity have led to criticism of the meta-analyses assessing pre-CRT for esophageal cancer,[29] which is also valid for trials assessing pre-CT. The survival and surgical outcomes from the individual RCTs including the most recent trial of pre-CT[7] are summarized in **Tables 1–3**.

Locally advanced esophageal cancer should be resected and the evidence supports the use of pre-CT or pre-CRT. Assessing the trials individually or using a meta-analysis does not offer a clear view of the optimal treatment of an individual.

What should an individual patient who presents with localized esophageal cancer be offered?

ISSUES TO BE CONSIDERED

The role of surgery and neoadjuvant therapy
- Aim to completely remove all known disease (R0 resection), so that recurrence, if it occurs, is systemic.
- Difficulties in widely resecting periesophageal tissues notably for tumors in the mid and upper esophagus.
- In Japanese centers, patients with SCC of the esophagus have the primary resected with a lymphadenectomy that includes abdominal, mediastinal and if relevant to the tumor site, cervical nodes (3-field dissection) to clear the regional disease.
- Recently, in Western countries, with a preponderance of AC in the lower esophagus, the trend is to clear the primary cancer along with the periesophageal, and the tissue around the celiac trunk in the abdomen (2-field lymph node dissection).
- Lymphatic drainage from the esophagus is more predictable for lesions in the lower esophagus and the EGJ when compared with the intrathoracic esophagus.[30]

- There is clear evidence for improved surgical outcomes in specialist centers performing a high volume of esophageal resections.[31,32]

The results from the surgery-alone arms, in the RCT, have been variable with respect to operative mortality and cancer survival. The RCTs between 1980 and 2000 were typically multicenter studies that included low-volume centers. These trials had little or no quality control over the surgery performed. A review of multimodality therapy for SCC of the esophagus, up to 1999,[33] reported the studies to have unreliable staging, the quality of the surgery was difficult to assess, and there was insufficient power in the RCTs. It was stated "unless uniform surgical therapy within a trial testing multimodality therapy is assured, any effect to determine the effects of other therapies is likely to be futile."

In the early trials, it is unlikely that aggressive locoregional resection occurred. There is indirect evidence for this observation when the margin status of the resected groups in the RCTs is examined (see **Tables 1** and **2**). In the early trials of pre-CT, the margins were clear in the surgery-alone group in 35% to 57% of patients with SCC. This finding improved to 44% to 71% after preoperative CT (see **Table 1**). For comparison, the most recent trials from Asia report excellent margin clearance in the surgery-alone arms,[1,7,34] with 2 trials reporting benefit, one from pre-CT[7] and the other pre-CRT.[1]

Trials from the West include AC of the lower esophagus and EGJAC as well as SCC. It is not possible to assess whether the site of the tumor has had an effect on the quality of the operation performed. Patients with AC have less association with major airways and major blood vessels, so the ability to achieve complete clearance of the cancer should be better than in patients with SCC in the mid and upper esophagus. Whether this difference has had an effect on trial outcomes is not clear.

The issue of survival outcomes in the surgery-alone arms of the RCTs has been examined. As the 2-year survival rates increased in the trials, the effect of the preoperative intervention decreased. At 2 years, the range of overall survival varied from 7% to 59%. This finding implies a differential absolute benefit for patients from the relevant neoadjuvant therapies. For example, in pre-CRT patients, if the 2-year survival was 20%, the number needed to treat (NNT) with pre-CRT, to save 1 life, was 7, but if the survival was 50%, the NNT was 10. From the pre-CT trials, if the 2-year survival was 20%, the NNT was 7, and if the survival was 50%, the NNT was 20.[35]

In a study assessing the outcome of patients who had pre-CRT, those considered fit to undergo

Table 1
CT then surgery versus surgery-alone trials: survival and surgical outcomes

Trial (Histology)	Trial Years (Number of Patients)	CT Cycles	Survival Median (mo)		Overall Survival		Locoregional Recurrence (%)		Margin Status Negative ITT (%)		Margin Status Negative After Surgery (%)		pCR (%)	Pathology Node Positive Status (%)	
			S	CS	S (%) (y)	CS (%)	S	CS	S	CS	S	CS	CS	S	CS
Roth et al,[13] 1988 (SCC)	1982–86 (36)	2 × Cis/vindesine/ bleomycin	9	9	5 3	25	n/s	—	21	35	21	35	6	n/s	—
Nygaard et al,[14] 1992 (SCC)	1983–88 (78)	2 × Cis/bleomycin	n/s	—	9 3	3	n/s	—	30	39	36	44	n/s	n/s	—
Schlag,[15] 1992 (SCC)	1980s (46)	3 × Cis/5FU	10	10	n/s	—	n/s	—	45	35	45	44	6	—	—
Maipang et al,[16] 1994 (SCC)	1988–90 (46)	2 × Cis/vinblastine bleomycin	12	17	36 3	31	n/s	—	n/s	—	n/s	—	n/s	n/s	—
Law et al,[17] 1997 (SCC)	1989–95 (147)	2 × Cis/5FU	13	17	31 2	44	30	12	33	54	35	67	7	88	70
Boonstra et al,[5] 2011 (SCC)	**1989–96 (169)**	**2 × Cis/etoposide**	**12**	**16**	**17 3**	**26**	**30**	**23**	**48**	**58**	**57**	**71**	**7**	**46**	**43**
Kelsen et al,[18] 2007 (AC 50%)	1990–95 (467)	3 × Cis/5FU	16	15	26 3	23	21	19	59	63	67	80	n/s	n/s	—
Ancona et al,[19] 2001 (SCC)	1992–97 (94)	3 × Cis/5FU[a]	24	25	22 5	34	34	32	79	74	87	90	13	n/s	—
Allum et al,[3] 2009 (AC 67%)	**1992–98 (802)**	**2 × Cis/5FU**	**13**	**17**	**17 5**	**23**	**12**	**12**	**53**	**58**	**65**	**69**	**4**	**68**	**58**
Ychou et al,[6] 2011 (AC 100%— 75% EGJ)[b]	1995–2003 (169)	2/3 × Cis/5FU	n/s	—	24 5	38	8	12	74	84	82	93	3	80	67
Ando et al,[7] 2012 (SCC)[c]	2000–06 (380)	2 × Cis/5FU	n/s	—	43 5	55	31[c]	25	89	90	91	95	2	76	65

Bold type = positive effect on overall survival from preoperative CT.
Locoregional recurrence = percentage of patients presenting with this site as first site of recurrence.
Abbreviations: 5FU, 5 fluorouracil; Cis, cisplatin; ITT, intention to treat; n/s, not stated; pCR, pathologic complete response after resection.
[a] Ancona and colleagues: 2 cycles of CT and then assessment of response. If present, a third cycle given (68%, 3 cycles).
[b] Patients with a response/stable disease or node positive after resection offered postoperative CT to a total of 6 cycles preoperatively and postoperatively.
[c] Postoperative CT offered to node-positive patients.
Data from Refs.[3,5–7,13–19]

Table 2
CRT then surgery versus surgery-alone trials: survival and surgical outcomes

Trial (Histology)	Trial Years (Number of Patients)	CT Cycles	Radiation Dose (Gy)	Survival Median (mo)		Overall Survival		Locoregional Recurrence (%)		Margin Status Negative ITT (%)		Margin Status Negative After Surgery (%)		pCR (%)	Pathology Node Positive Status (%)	
				S	CRT	S (%) (y)	CRT (%)	S	CRT	S	CRT	S	CRT	CRT	S	CRT
Nygaard et al,[14] 1992 (SCC)	1983–88 (78)	2 × Cis/Etop	35	n/s	n/s	9 3	17	n/s	—	30	49	36	55	n/s	38	29
Apinop et al,[20] 1994 (SCC)	1986–92 (69)	2 × Cis/5FU	40	7	10	10 5	24	n/s	—	n/s	—	n/s	—	n/s	n/s	—
Le Prise et al,[21] 1994 (SCC)	1988–91 (86)	2 × Cis/5FU	20	n/s	n/s	14 3	19	20	17	n/s	—	n/s	—	10	55	38
Bosset et al,[23] 1997 (SCC)	1989–95 (293)	2 × Cis	37	19	19	35 3	37	n/s	—	68	78	69	81	—	55	38
Walsh,[24] 1995 (AC)	**1990–95 (113)**	**2 × Cis/5FU**	**40**	**11**	**16**	**6 3**	**32**	**n/s**	—	**n/s**	—	**n/s**	—	**22**	**82**	**42**
Urba et al,[22] 2001 (AC 75%)	1989–94 (293)	2 × Cis/5FU/Vin	45	18	17	12 5	20	42	19	88	88	98	98	28	n/s	—

Study	Years (n)	Regimen															
Burmeister et al,[25] 2005 (AC 62%)	1994–2000 (256)	1 × Cis/5FU	35	19	22	33	3	33	14	11	59	81	69	100	13	67	43
Tepper et al,[9] 2008 (AC 75%)	**1997–2000 (56)**	**2 × Cis/5FU**	**50.4**	**22**	**53**	**16**	**5**	**39**	**11**	**3**	**n/s**	**—**	**n/s**	**—**	**33**	**n/s**	**—**
Lv et al,[1] 2010 (SCC)[a]	**1997–2004 (160)**	**2 × Cis/ placitaxel**	**40**	**36**	**53**	**34**	**5**	**44**	**35**	**11**	**80**	**97**	**83**	**100**	**n/s**	**n/s**	**—**
Lee et al,[34] 2004 (SCC)[b]	1999–2002 (101)	2 × Cis/5FU	45.6	27	28	57	2	55	12	22	84	69	91	100	43	78	37
Mariette et al,[26] 2010 (SCC 70%)[c]	2000–09 (195)	2 × Cis/5FU	45	44	32	55	3	49	n/s	—	86	88	n/s	—	n/s	n/s	—
van Hagen et al,[10] 2012 (AC 75%)	**2004–08 (364)**	**5 × carboplatin/ placitaxel**	**41.4**	**24**	**49**	**34**	**5**	**47**	**n/s**	**—**	**59**	**82**	**69**	**92**	**26**	**75**	**31**

Bold = positive effect on overall survival from preoperative chemoradiation.

Locoregional recurrence = percentage of patients presenting with this site as first site of recurrence.

Abbreviations: 5FU, 5 fluorouracil; Carbo, carboplatin; Cis, cisplatin; Etop, etoposide; ITT, intention to treat; n/s, not stated; pCR, pathologic complete response after resection; Vin, vindesine.

[a] Three-arm trial: pre-CRT versus surgery alone versus post-CRT: same CT preoperatively and postoperatively.

[b] Patients who had resection and had a disease response or the disease was stable were offered 3 cycles Cis/5FU (60% patients).

[c] Included patients with early-stage disease – T1/T2 – 41% patients.

Data from Refs.[1,8–10,14,20–23,25,26,34]

Table 3
CRT then surgery versus CT then surgery trials: survival and surgical outcomes

Trial (Histology)	Trial Years (Number of Patients)	CT Cycles	Radiation Dose (Gy)	Survival Median (mo)		Overall Survival		Locoregional Recurrence (%)		Margin Status Negative ITT (%)		Margin Status Negative After Surgery (%)		pCR (%)		Pathology Node Positive Status (%)	
				CS	CRT	CS (%) (y)	CRT (%)	CS	CRT	CS	CRT	CS	CRT	CS	CRT	CS	CRT
Burmeister et al,[28] 2005 (AC)	2000–2006 (72)	2 × Cis/5FU vs 2 × Cis/5FU	35	29	32	36 5	45	11	8	81	85	88	100	0	13	n/s	—
Stahl et al,[27] 2009 (AC)	2000–2005 (119)	3 × Cis/5FU/Leu vs 2.5 × Cis/5FU/Leu	30	21	33	28 3	47	24	15	69	72	79	88	2	12	63	36

Locoregional recurrence = percentage of patients presenting with this site as first site of recurrence.
Abbreviations: 5FU, 5 fluorouracil; Cis, cisplatin; Leu, leucovorin; ITT, intention to treat; n/s, not stated; pCR, pathologic complete response after resection.
Data from Refs.[27,28]

an en bloc esophagectomy were compared with patients who were less robust or for other reasons had a transhiatal esophagectomy. There was a better survival in the patients who had the more radical surgery independent of an excellent response to the pre-CRT or lack of response. The conclusion was that the extent of the operation had an impact.[36] In a study of patients with SCC who had pre-CRT,[37] the degree of lymph node dissection did not influence the overall survival in patients who had a complete pathologic response (cPR). In patients without a cPR, an inadequate lymph node dissection adversely affected survival,[37] suggesting that the quality of the surgery is important, especially for nonresponders.

Overall, the quality of the operation is an important component in the treatment of the patient who presents with esophageal cancer. The presence of poor outcomes in the control arms of gastrointestinal surgical trials was recently highlighted, with recommendations that reviewers and investigators of meta-analyses should evaluate carefully whether the outcomes in trials are consistent with contemporary publications.[38] In the trials of neoadjuvant therapy for esophageal cancer, it may be that the preoperative therapy was not the only variable affecting outcome in several of the trials, notably those performed before 2000.

Induction (neoadjuvant) CT (see **Table 1**)
- Treats occult metastatic disease.
- After pre-CT, a major effect on the primary cancer or overt nodal disease would not be expected. If that effect happens, it is a bonus.
- Preoperative CT needs to be followed by adequate surgery for the locoregional management of the disease.
- Typical pre-CT regimens include cisplatin and 5 fluorouracil (5FU).
- Recently, taxanes have been validated in the management of esophageal cancer in combination with radiotherapy, particularly paclitaxel.[1,10,39,40] These taxanes have not been tested in pre-CT regimens without radiotherapy.
- Outcomes between a lower esophageal cancer and EGJ cancer are not significantly different when adjusted for stage.[41,42]
- There is evidence for a difference between cancer at the gastric cardia/EGJ and noncardia cancer,[43,44] which may be relevant in recent Western trials.

A Cochrane review of studies before 2000 reported a 2-year difference in cancer mortality of 20% in patients having pre-CT (odds ratio = 0.80; 95% confidence interval 0.65–0.99). In years 3 to 5, the outcomes favored pre-CT, but the

confidence intervals were not significant.[45] The early RCTs assessing the effect of pre-CT, in patients with SCC, were small, underpowered, had poor staging, and poor surgery-alone outcomes. Despite this situation, there were patients who responded to CT, and there was some improvement in the surgical outcomes from the therapy (see **Table 1**).

The 2 largest pre-CT trials were performed during the same timeline, from 1992 to 1998. The UK trial[3] used 2 cycles of cisplatin and 5FU, and the US trial[18] used the same drugs but with 3 cycles. The UK trial reported a positive effect from pre-CT, but the US trial was negative. These studies had a mixed population of patients with SCC and AC and the surgery was performed in multiple centers. Possible reasons for the conflicting results include the delay to definitive surgery in the US trial (median 63 vs 93 days), more patients in the UK trial had a resection (92% vs 80%), the US trial included more patients with stage I and II disease, and half the patients in the US trial received at least 1 cycle of CT postoperatively.

However, despite the conflicting outcomes in those 2 trials, the most recent pre-CT trials report positive outcomes. Two were in Western countries involving patients with AC. Both studies included patients with gastric cancer, although to varying degrees. A UK trial[46] included 26% of patients with AC at the EGJ (11.5%) or in the lower esophagus (14.5%). Patients received 3 cycles of epirubicin, cisplatin, and 5FU preoperatively and after resection. Postoperative CT was completed in 42% of patients. The 5-year survival for the perioperative CT group was 36% compared with 23% for the surgery-alone group. In a French trial,[6] 75% of patients had cancer at the EGJ (64%) or lower esophagus (11%), and the patients received 2 to 3 cycles of cisplatin and 5FU preoperatively. A further 3 to 4 cycles were offered postoperatively to a total of 6 cycles. The 5-year survival for the treated patients was 38% compared with 24% in surgery-alone patients. Despite the difference in sites, the survival figures are similar. The delay to surgery, because of a third cycle of CT in these trials, has not had a detrimental influence, which was proposed as 1 reason for the US trial being negative. The impact of the heterogeneity of the trials with respect to the site of tumor is not clear. Nevertheless, there seems to be a benefit from the use of perioperative CT in patients with AC of the esophagus and EGJ, which was not clearly seen from the very early pre-CT trials for SCC in Western studies.

The third positive trial was performed in Japan[7] and was not included in the recent meta-analysis. Patients with SCC had 2 cycles of cisplatin and 5FU followed by surgery. Postoperatively, cisplatin and 5FU were offered to patients who were node positive. The 5-year survival rate in both arms is the highest of all the pre-CT trials (see **Table 1**).

Thus, there is evidence for pre-CT in patients with AC. For patients with SCC, using Western trial data, the evidence is not so strong; however, this may relate to the period in which the trials were performed, given the outcome from the recent Japanese report. In patients having pre-CT (without RT), surgery is the only means of local therapy, so the quality of the surgery is likely to be an important variable.

Neoadjuvant CRT (see **Table 2**)

- Evidence for the benefit of the addition of CT to a radiation dose of 50.4 Gy for definitive management of esophageal cancer in a trial with predominately SCC (88%)[47] stimulated the use of similar regimens in a preoperative setting.
- Higher doses of radiation when used for definitive therapy showed no improvement in survival or locoregional control.[48]
- May reduce or eradicate the primary cancer.
- Improves the rate of complete resection of the cancer.
- There is no clear information on appropriate dose of radiotherapy in the neoadjuvant setting.
- Most trials have used the combination of cisplatin and 5 FU concurrent with the radiation.
- Recent evidence to support the use of the taxanes and platinum derivatives.
- Evidence supports a minimum of 2 cycles of CT when used with radiotherapy, with no data on optimal number of cycles of CT.

In the pre-CRT trials, little to no effect from the treatment was seen when patients had a single cycle of CT,[25] sequential CT,[21,23] or when there were many early-stage patients.[26]

There are 4 positive studies, 2 with patients with mixed histology (AC 75%)[9,10] and 1 each with AC alone[8] and SCC alone.[1] The 2 older studies reported 5-year survivals in the control arms of less than 20%.[8,9]

The most recent study reports a benefit with a 5-year survival of 47% compared with 34% for the surgery-alone group. Patients received 5 cycles of the combination of paclitaxel and carboplatin with 41.4 Gy radiation concurrent with the last cycle. Patients had modern staging with computed tomography and endoscopic ultrasonographic (EUS) assessment, allowing better stage stratification and definition of surgery requirements. A transhiatal approach was used for the lower third

cancers (80% of cases). A positive effect was seen in patients with AC and SCC, with the effect appearing larger in the SCC group, although the numbers were small.[10]

A trial of patients with SCC, from South Korea,[1] had a third arm of postoperative CRT. Paclitaxel and cisplatin were given in 2 cycles with concurrent 40 Gy radiotherapy during the second cycle. The 5-year survival from the pre-CRT was 44% compared with 34% in the surgery-alone arm. There was a similar advantage in survival from postoperative CRT, with no difference between the preoperative and postoperative therapy arms.

From 2 reviews of pre-CRT over 2 different periods,[49,50] there was no agreement on dose and scheduling for both CT and radiotherapy. The latest review assessed patients treated from 2000 to 2008.[50] The mortality related from the CRT treatment was 2.7%. Most of the pre-CRT studies have used a radiation dose of 45 Gy, with a major focus on tumor response and complete clearance of the primary tumor. In the RCTs, the radiation doses varied from 20 to 50.4 Gy (see **Table 2**). In the latest review, the average percentage of patients who had a resection was 83.6%. The mean complete resection rate (R0) from 23 studies was 88.4%, and the pCR rate ranged between 13% and 49% (mean 25.8%). Patients who had a pCR have a better overall survival than nonresponders.[50]

Overall, there is evidence for the use of pre-CRT in patients with AC and SCC. The added value radiotherapy offers with respect to pCR and margin clearance when compared with pre-CT is worthy of debate, considering that radiation is a local therapy and that the most common cause of death in these patients is distant metastasis. In addition, there is evidence for increased anastomotic complications at the higher doses of preoperative radiotherapy.[51] The question is how much benefit, if any, does radiotherapy offer above pre-CT when a patient has appropriate surgery for the primary cancer and the regional nodes?

Pre-CT compared with pre-CRT (see **Table 3**)

- There are no adequately powered trials to address this question.
- Typically, centers have policies related to local issues and potential specialty biases.

A recent single-institution study retrospectively analyzed patients who were recruited to phase 2 and 3 trials involving pre-CT and pre-CRT. The cohort who received preoperative CT over 1 period (1990–1995) were compared with another who received preoperative CRT over a later period (1996–2000); reported survival outcomes were higher in the pre-CRT group (5 years = 31%) compared with pre-CT group (5 years = 21%). However, the CRT group had more postoperative complications and the operative mortality was 7% compared with 4% for the CT group (not significant).[52] In a cohort study such as this, one needs to be wary of drawing major conclusions. Only 75% of the patients in the CT group compared with 90% in the CRT group had a resection. Also, the issue of better staging and selection for surgery is likely to be real, given the 2 periods.

There are 2 small trials that have formally examined the question of pre-CT versus pre-CRT. Both used the same CT in each arm, with radiotherapy being the variable assessed in the randomization.[27,28] Both studies were underpowered and were assessed together in the latest meta-analysis.[12] Just as there are problems assessing the other RCT in the meta-analysis, there are problems combining these studies. Although both studies focused on AC and were performed at the same period, the German trial was multicentered and 15% of the patients had a total gastrectomy. The Australian study was a single-unit trial and all patients had a formal esophagogastrectomy with abdominal and chest approaches by experienced surgeons in a high-volume center. In the German study, the outcomes in the pre-CT arm, including survival, locoregional recurrence and complete resection status, were worse than the Australian study. The outcomes in the pre-CRT arms were similar. The Australian study was negative and the German study reported a nonsignificant trend for preoperative CRT to be superior. This was also the conclusion when the trials were combined (192 patients) in the recent meta-analysis.[12] Whether there is a real difference between the 2 treatments in the environment of appropriate surgery is not clear.

SPECIFIC ISSUES

The role of complete pathologic response (cPR)
- Patients who have cPR after pre-CRT have a better prognosis than a lesser response.[53–56]
- cPR after pre-CT is associated with an improved survival compared with nonresponders.[13,17,18,57]
- Major response after pre-CRT, less than 10% of viable residual cancer,[56] offers a better prognosis than lesser responses.[58]
- pCR rates, after pre-CRT, vary from 13% to 49%, with no clear relationship with histology, radiation dose, the CT agents (up to 2010), and the timing of the resection after completion of CRT.[50]

- pCR rates increase with higher total radiation dose, shorter treatment time, lower age, and higher CT dose.[59]
- pCR rates are higher after pre-CRT than pre-CT (see **Tables 1–3**).

The highest pCR rate in all the RCTs (43%) was achieved with hyperfractionated radiotherapy (45.6 Gy) in a Korean study of patients with SCC.[34] This trial reported no benefit from pre-CRT. Postoperatively, those who had a pathologic response or stable disease on pathology were offered CT (60% of the resected group). The 2 recent trials reporting a survival benefit from preoperative CRT had pCR rates of 33%[9] and 26%.[10] Both trials included patients with AC and SCC. The trial from the CALGB (Cancer and Leukemia Group B) had 28 patients in the treatment arm scheduled to receive a radiotherapy dose of 50.5 Gy (the highest dose used in the CRT trials). The Netherlands study had 178 patients scheduled to receive a radiotherapy dose of 41.4 Gy. When assessing cancer survival, in these studies, the 2-year survival (from the survival curves) in the CALGB trial was 70% and in the Netherlands trial, 67%, compared with 55% for the Korean study (highest pCR rate). The 5-year survivals, from the 2 positive trials, were 39% and 49%, respectively. The Netherlands study used a different regimen of CT from the CALGB study, yet the results were similar.

For comparison, the 2 trials comparing preoperative CRT with CT, in patients with AC, used radiotherapy doses of 35 Gy[28] and 30 Gy,[27] with concurrent cycles of cisplatin and 5FU. Despite low pCR rates of 13%[28] and 12%,[27] the 2-year and 5-year survivals were 66%/45%[28] and 67%/47%,[27] similar to the previous reports in patients who had higher radiotherapy doses and better pCR rates.

In the pre-CT trials, it is no surprise that without the local effect of radiotherapy, the cPR in the resected specimens were as low as 0% to 7% (see **Table 1**). However, despite the low pCR rates, there was a positive effect on overall survival in several trials.[3,5–7]

The addition of radiotherapy to pre-CT is seen as a more attractive option than pre-CT alone, because of the higher pCR rates. It has been stated that "high pCR is a prerequisite for long term survival."[34] A significant primary tumor response to neoadjuvant therapy is a biological marker in the cohorts studied, relevant for pre-CT and pre-CRT. The addition of radiotherapy for local treatment of the cancer offers an increased assessment of the biology of the cancer but remains a local therapy. In a study of patients with

AC who had an esophagectomy and a lymphade-nectomy with more than 18 nodes removed, pre-CRT had no effect on the overall or disease-specific survival.[60] A recent study reported that pCR was not synonymous with cure or complete local control and in a multivariate model of variables predicting cancer survival, the post pre-CRT lymph node status was the only independent factor that was positive.[54]

There is no clear evidence that increasing the pCR rate clearly influences the end point of overall survival in the whole cohort of patients treated. It would be more realistic to consider the research focus on increasing pCR as part of the paradigm of avoidance of an esophagectomy. Alternatively, assessing response to neoadjuvant therapy may stratify therapies focusing on the poorer prognostic nonresponders. Thus, methods that assess primary tumor response to pre-CT and pre-CRT are important research themes because prediction of primary tumor response or evidence may allow a more personalized approach to therapy.

If the tumor is completely removed, the most important outcome is cancer survival, not pCR rate.

Complete resection of the cancer (R0): margin and node status after neoadjuvant therapy
- The circumferential margin of the primary cancer is the most likely site to be involved after an esophagectomy.
- Margin involvement occurs because of inadequate surgical clearance for technical reasons or because of the extent of the primary tumor, relating to tumor biology.
- The margin status after an esophageal resection has been shown, in cohort studies, to be an independent prognostic factor in the cancer outcomes in patients who have pre-CRT[61] and pre-CT.[62]

If resection margins reported in cohort studies are compared with those reported in RCTs, the outcomes need to be carefully assessed. In cohort studies, patients considered for resection and who commenced therapy, but did not have an operation or who had a palliative resection (R2), were often excluded from the analysis. In the RCTs, there are patients randomized who do not have resection (more in the neoadjuvant therapy arms than the surgery-alone arms). Thus, outcomes reported on an intention-to-treat (ITT) basis compared with resected groups are different (see **Tables 1–3**).

Before 2000, in the RCTs, the surgery-alone arms reported clear margins in less than 70% of patients in all but 1 study (see **Tables 1** and **2**). The more recent studies have reported higher clearance rates in the surgery-alone arms. As expected, pre-CRT improves the margin status (see **Table 2**). In the pre-CT studies, notably in the early trials, which involved patients with SCC, the margin status was improved both on ITT and in patients who had a resection, implying a local effect from the CT. The more recent preoperative CT studies have reported an improvement in margin status in general without an effect from the pre-CT (see **Table 1**). The recent changes in margin status in all of the trials in the surgery-alone arms may relate to technical issues as well as better patient staging and selection for trial inclusion.

Examining the primary tumor characteristics, the T3 and T4 cancers have the potential for radial margin involvement. When focusing on this T-stage subset, a positive margin in a patient having appropriate surgery has a prognostic impact[62]; however, the impact from the margin status on overall survival is questionable.[63] Although the sensitivity of preoperative EUS is poor in differentiating T1 and T2 primary tumors, the sensitivity is as high as 91% in defining T1/T2 compared with T3/T4 tumors.[64] EUS can be used as an important tool in defining which patient should have neoadjuvant therapy and also which therapy may be appropriate.

It is reasonable to consider that the lymph node status after resection may affect outcome in a patient who has had preoperative therapy. When reported, in both the pre-CT trials and the pre-CRT trials, there is a reduction in the number of patients with positive lymph nodes (see **Tables 1** and **2**). The effect is highest in the pre-CRT trials. The largest change reported was a 44% reduction,[10] with others reporting slightly lower figures[8,34] and 2 of these trials reporting a survival benefit from the CRT.[8,10] In the CT trials, there was also a reduction in positive lymph nodes (3%–23%). Although to a lesser degree than pre-CRT, a positive survival effect from the pre-CT was reported in these trials.[3,5–7]

If the patient has had an appropriate resection, a positive margin is likely to represent a biological marker of more aggressive and infiltrative disease. If cancer survival is the major end point, in a patient who is having appropriate surgery, the extra benefit to overall survival by the addition of radiotherapy to pre-CT is not clear.

LOCOREGIONAL CONTROL

Locoregional control, once resection has been performed, is an important end point with this disease. In assessing the incidence of isolated locoregional recurrence, the outcomes are variable. For patients having pre-CT, there was no significant difference when compared with surgery alone (see **Table 1**). In patients having

Table 4
Active RCTs (phase 3) of neoadjuvant therapy for esophageal cancer

Country	Trial Name	Histology	Treatment	Number	Primary End Point	Status
United Kingdom (MRC)	OEO5	AC/EGJ	Cis/5FU × 2 surgery vs Epi/Cis/Xel × 4 surgery	1300	Overall survival	Closed 2011 Analysis late 2013
United Kingdom (MRC)	STO3	AC Gastric/Esophageal/EGJ[a]	Epi/Cis/Xel × 3 surgery vs Epi/Cis/Xel/Bev surgery	1100	Overall survival	Open Initially gastric Lately recruiting lower esophageal and EGJ[a]
Sweden/Norway	NeoRes	AC SCC Esophageal/EGJ	Cis/5FU × 3 surgery vs Cis/5FU RT = 40 Gy surgery	180	CPR rates	Closed early 2013
Japan (JCOG)	NExT (JCOG 1109)	SCC	Cis/5FU × 2 surgery vs Doc/Cis/5FU × 3 surgery vs Cis/5FU × 2 RT = 41.4 Gy surgery	501	Overall survival	Commenced December 2012

Abbreviations: Cis, cisplatin; Doc, docetaxel; Epi, epirubicin; JCOG, Japanese Clinical Oncology Group; MRC, Medical Research Council; Xel, Xeloda (capcitabine).
[a] Originally restricted to gastric cancer. With closure of OEO5, patients now recruited to STO3 similar to the previous MAGIC trial (Cunningham and colleagues[46]).

preoperative CRT, there was a significant reduction in 2 trials (see **Table 2**),[1,22] but no effect on overall cancer survival. There was no difference in the 2 trials that compared preoperative CT with CRT (see **Table 3**). Patients having pCR from pre-CRT have less isolated local recurrence rates, but this does not affect the cancer survival.[54]

FUTURE RCTS

Table 4 summarizes the trials that have just been completed or that are actively assessing neoadjuvant therapy for esophageal cancer. The study in Japan is important in that it focuses on patients with SCC only and has 3 arms examining 2 protocols of pre-CT and a third arm of pre-CRT. Patients will have standardized surgery. The Medical Research Council trial, OEO5, in the United Kingdom will offer an insight into the role of epirubicin in pre-CT. With the closure of OEO5, patients are now recruiting to the STO3 trial, in which the role of the biological targeted therapy, bevacizumab, will be assessed in patients with AC.

The Swedish trial will add to the literature on pre-CRT compared with pre-CT but will not address the issue of cancer survival, given the small numbers being recruited.

SUMMARY

- Neoadjuvant therapy with CT or CRT improves survival in patients with locally advanced esophageal cancer.
- There is no robust study that has directly compared neoadjuvant CT with neoadjuvant CRT for patients with SCC or AC.
- The results of at least 3 trials are awaited to provide further information on which CT should be offered and more information on the role of the addition of radiotherapy to pre-CT.

So for the individual patient

No one treatment fits all.
The decision should be based on histology, local staging using EUS along with local and systemic staging with computed tomography/fluorodeoxyglucose positron emission tomography.
For an invasive carcinoma, patients should have pre-CT.
Consider the addition of radiation to pre-CT when the patient has a locally advanced carcinoma that is T3 and it is likely that surgery will not completely remove the tumor.
The decision relating to the ability to resect may include considerations such as the association of the primary cancer with major anatomic structures.

Future

The future will involve the assessment of newer chemotherapeutic agents that have a greater effect on occult disease. It is likely that research into the molecular basis of cancer of the esophagus will offer insights into selection of specific therapeutic options for an individual based on the genetics of the primary tumor along with responses that occur to CT or CRT.

REFERENCES

1. Lv J, Cao XF, Zhu B, et al. Long-term efficacy of perioperative chemoradiotherapy on esophageal squamous cell carcinoma. World J Gastroenterol 2010;16(13):1649–54.
2. Arnott SJ, Duncan W, Gignoux M, et al. Preoperative radiotherapy for esophageal carcinoma. Cochrane Database Syst Rev 2005;(4):CD001799.
3. Allum WH, Stenning SP, Bancewicz J, et al. Long-term results of a randomized trial of surgery with or without preoperative chemotherapy in esophageal cancer. J Clin Oncol 2009;27(30):5062–7.
4. Medical Research Council Oesophageal Cancer Working Group. Surgical resection with or without preoperative chemotherapy in oesophageal cancer: a randomised controlled trial. Lancet 2002; 359(9319):1727–33.
5. Boonstra JJ, Kok TC, Wijnhoven BP, et al. Chemotherapy followed by surgery versus surgery alone in patients with resectable oesophageal squamous cell carcinoma: long-term results of a randomized controlled trial. BMC Cancer 2011;11:181.
6. Ychou M, Boige V, Pignon JP, et al. Perioperative chemotherapy compared with surgery alone for resectable gastroesophageal adenocarcinoma: an FNCLCC and FFCD multicenter phase III trial. J Clin Oncol 2011;29(13):1715–21.
7. Ando N, Kato H, Igaki H, et al. A randomized trial comparing postoperative adjuvant chemotherapy with cisplatin and 5-fluorouracil versus preoperative chemotherapy for localized advanced squamous cell carcinoma of the thoracic esophagus (JCOG9907). Ann Surg Oncol 2012;19(1):68–74.
8. Walsh TN, Noonan N, Hollywood D, et al. A comparison of multimodal therapy and surgery for esophageal adenocarcinoma. N Engl J Med 1996;335(7): 462–7.
9. Tepper J, Krasna MJ, Niedzwiecki D, et al. Phase III trial of trimodality therapy with cisplatin, fluorouracil, radiotherapy, and surgery compared with surgery alone for esophageal cancer: CALGB 9781. J Clin Oncol 2008;26(7):1086–92.

10. van Hagen P, Hulshof MC, van Lanschot JJ, et al. Preoperative chemoradiotherapy for esophageal or junctional cancer. N Engl J Med 2012;366(22): 2074–84.

11. Iyer R, Wilkinson N, Demmy T, et al. Controversies in the multimodality management of locally advanced esophageal cancer: evidence-based review of surgery alone and combined-modality therapy. Ann Surg Oncol 2004;11(7):665–73.

12. Sjoquist KM, Burmeister BH, Smithers BM, et al. Survival after neoadjuvant chemotherapy or chemoradiotherapy for resectable oesophageal carcinoma: an updated meta-analysis. Lancet Oncol 2011;12(7):681–92.

13. Roth JA, Pass HI, Flanagan MM, et al. Randomized clinical trial of preoperative and postoperative adjuvant chemotherapy with cisplatin, vindesine, and bleomycin for carcinoma of the esophagus. J Thorac Cardiovasc Surg 1988;96(2):242–8.

14. Nygaard K, Hagen S, Hansen HS, et al. Pre-operative radiotherapy prolongs survival in operable esophageal carcinoma: a randomized, multicenter study of pre-operative radiotherapy and chemotherapy. The second Scandinavian trial in esophageal cancer. World J Surg 1992;16(6):1104–9 [discussion: 1110].

15. Schlag PM. Randomized trial of preoperative chemotherapy for squamous cell cancer of the esophagus. The Chirurgische Arbeitsgemeinschaft fuer Onkologie der Deutschen Gesellschaft fuer Chirurgie Study Group. Arch Surg 1992;127(12): 1446–50.

16. Maipang T, Vasinanukorn P, Petpichetchian C, et al. Induction chemotherapy in the treatment of patients with carcinoma of the esophagus. J Surg Oncol 1994;56(3):191–7.

17. Law S, Fok M, Chow S, et al. Preoperative chemotherapy versus surgical therapy alone for squamous cell carcinoma of the esophagus: a prospective randomized trial. J Thorac Cardiovasc Surg 1997; 114(2):210–7.

18. Kelsen DP, Winter KA, Gunderson LL, et al. Long-term results of RTOG trial 8911 (USA Intergroup 113): a random assignment trial comparison of chemotherapy followed by surgery compared with surgery alone for esophageal cancer. J Clin Oncol 2007;25(24):3719–25.

19. Ancona E, Ruol A, Santi S, et al. Only pathologic complete response to neoadjuvant chemotherapy improves significantly the long term survival of patients with resectable esophageal squamous cell carcinoma: final report of a randomized, controlled trial of preoperative chemotherapy versus surgery alone. Cancer 2001;91(11):2165–74.

20. Apinop C, Puttisak P, Preecha N. A prospective study of combined therapy in esophageal cancer. Hepatogastroenterology 1994;41(4):391–3.

21. Le Prise E, Etienne PL, Meunier B, et al. A randomized study of chemotherapy, radiation therapy, and surgery versus surgery for localized squamous cell carcinoma of the esophagus. Cancer 1994;73(7):1779–84.

22. Urba SG, Orringer MB, Turrisi A, et al. Randomized trial of preoperative chemoradiation versus surgery alone in patients with locoregional esophageal carcinoma. J Clin Oncol 2001;19(2):305–13.

23. Bosset JF, Gignoux M, Triboulet JP, et al. Chemoradiotherapy followed by surgery compared with surgery alone in squamous-cell cancer of the esophagus. N Engl J Med 1997;337(3):161–7.

24. Walsh T. The role of multimodality therapy in improving survival: a prospective randomised trial [MD thesis]. In: Predicting, defining and improving outcomes for oesophageal carcinoma. Dublin (Ireland): Trinity College, University of Dublin; 1995. p. 124–50.

25. Burmeister BH, Smithers BM, Gebski V, et al. Surgery alone versus chemoradiotherapy followed by surgery for resectable cancer of the oesophagus: a randomised controlled phase III trial. Lancet Oncol 2005;6(9):659–68.

26. Mariette C, Seitz JF, Maillard E, et al, Federation Francaise de Cancerologie Digestive. Surgery alone versus chemoradiotherapy followed by surgery for localized esophageal cancer: analysis of a randomized controlled phase III trial FFCD 9901. J Clin Oncol Proc Am Soc Clin Oncol 2010; 28(15) [abstract 4005].

27. Stahl M, Walz MK, Stuschke M, et al. Phase III comparison of preoperative chemotherapy compared with chemoradiotherapy in patients with locally advanced adenocarcinoma of the esophagogastric junction. J Clin Oncol 2009;27(6):851–6.

28. Burmeister BH, Thomas JM, Burmeister EA, et al. Is concurrent radiation therapy required in patients receiving preoperative chemotherapy for adenocarcinoma of the oesophagus? A randomised phase II trial. Eur J Cancer 2011;47(3):354–60.

29. Wijnhoven BP, van Lanschot JJ, Tilanus HW, et al. Neoadjuvant chemoradiotherapy for esophageal cancer: a review of meta-analyses. World J Surg 2009;33(12):2606–14.

30. Stein HJ, Feith M, Bruecher BL, et al. Early esophageal cancer: pattern of lymphatic spread and prognostic factors for long-term survival after surgical resection. Ann Surg 2005;242(4):566–73 [discussion: 573–5].

31. Metzger R, Bollschweiler E, Vallbohmer D, et al. High volume centers for esophagectomy: what is the number needed to achieve low postoperative mortality? Dis Esophagus 2004;17(4):310–4.

32. Rouvelas I, Lagergren J. The impact of volume on outcomes after oesophageal cancer surgery. ANZ J Surg 2010;80(9):634–41.

33. Lehnert T. Multimodal therapy for squamous carcinoma of the oesophagus. Br J Surg 1999;86(6):727–39.

34. Lee JL, Park SI, Kim SB, et al. A single institutional phase III trial of preoperative chemotherapy with hyperfractionation radiotherapy plus surgery versus surgery alone for resectable esophageal squamous cell carcinoma. Ann Oncol 2004;15(6):947–54.

35. Gebski V, Burmeister B, Smithers BM, et al. Survival benefits from neoadjuvant chemoradiotherapy or chemotherapy in oesophageal carcinoma: a meta-analysis. Lancet Oncol 2007;8(3):226–34.

36. Rizzetto C, DeMeester SR, Hagen JA, et al. En bloc esophagectomy reduces local recurrence and improves survival compared with transhiatal resection after neoadjuvant therapy for esophageal adenocarcinoma. J Thorac Cardiovasc Surg 2008;135(6):1228–36.

37. Chao YK, Liu HP, Hsieh MJ, et al. Lymph node dissection after chemoradiation in esophageal cancer: a subgroup analysis of patients with and without pathological response. Ann Surg Oncol 2012;19(11):3500–5.

38. Strobel O, Buchler MW. The problem of the poor control arm in surgical randomized controlled trials. Br J Surg 2013;100(2):172–3.

39. Jimenez P, Pathak A, Phan AT. The role of taxanes in the management of gastroesophageal cancer. J Gastrointest Oncol 2011;2(4):240–9.

40. Gannett DE, Wolf RF, Takahashi GW, et al. Neoadjuvant chemoradiotherapy for esophageal cancer using weekly paclitaxel and carboplatin plus infusional 5-fluorouracil. Gastrointest Cancer Res 2007;1(4):132–8.

41. Portale G, Peters JH, Hagen JA, et al. Comparison of the clinical and histological characteristics and survival of distal esophageal-gastroesophageal junction adenocarcinoma in patients with and without Barrett mucosa. Arch Surg 2005;140:570–5.

42. Wijnhoven BP, Siersema PD, Hop WC, et al. Adenocarcinomas of the distal oesophagus and gastric cardia are one clinical entity. Rotterdam Oesophageal Tumour Study Group. Br J Surg 1999;86(4):529–35.

43. Rohde H, Bauer P, Stutzer H, et al. Proximal compared with distal adenocarcinoma of the stomach: differences and consequences. German Gastric Cancer TNM Study Group. Br J Surg 1991;78(10):1242–8.

44. Heidl G, Langhans P, Mellin W, et al. Adenocarcinomas of esophagus and cardia in comparison with gastric carcinoma. J Cancer Res Clin Oncol 1993;120(1–2):95–9.

45. Malthaner R, Fenton D. Preoperative chemotherapy for resectable thoracic esophageal cancer. Cochrane Database Syst Rev 2002;1.

46. Cunningham D, Allum WH, Stenning SP, et al. Perioperative chemotherapy versus surgery alone for resectable gastroesophageal cancer. N Engl J Med 2006;355(1):11–20.

47. Herskovic A, Martz K, al-Sarraf M, et al. Combined chemotherapy and radiotherapy compared with radiotherapy alone in patients with cancer of the esophagus. N Engl J Med 1992;326(24):1593–8.

48. Minsky BD, Pajak TF, Ginsberg RJ, et al. INT 0123 (Radiation Therapy Oncology Group 94-05) phase III trial of combined-modality therapy for esophageal cancer: high-dose versus standard-dose radiation therapy. J Clin Oncol 2002;20(5):1167–74.

49. Geh JI, Crellin AM, Glynne-Jones R. Preoperative (neoadjuvant) chemoradiotherapy in oesophageal cancer. Br J Surg 2001;88(3):338–56.

50. Courrech Staal EF, Aleman BM, Boot H, et al. Systematic review of the benefits and risks of neoadjuvant chemoradiation for oesophageal cancer. Br J Surg 2010;97(10):1482–96.

51. Vande Walle C, Ceelen WP, Boterberg T, et al. Anastomotic complications after Ivor Lewis esophagectomy in patients treated with neoadjuvant chemoradiation are related to radiation dose to the gastric fundus. Int J Radiat Oncol Biol Phys 2012;82(3):e513–9.

52. Swisher SG, Hofstetter W, Komaki R, et al. Improved long-term outcome with chemoradiotherapy strategies in esophageal cancer. Ann Thorac Surg 2010;90(3):892–8 [discussion: 898–9].

53. Brucher BL, Weber W, Bauer M, et al. Neoadjuvant therapy of esophageal squamous cell carcinoma: response evaluation by positron emission tomography. Ann Surg 2001;233(3):300–9.

54. van Hagen P, Wijnhoven BP, Nafteux P, et al. Recurrence pattern in patients with a pathologically complete response after neoadjuvant chemoradiotherapy and surgery for oesophageal cancer. Br J Surg 2013;100(2):267–73.

55. Schneider PM, Baldus SE, Metzger R, et al. Histomorphologic tumor regression and lymph node metastases determine prognosis following neoadjuvant radiochemotherapy for esophageal cancer: implications for response classification. Ann Surg 2005;242(5):684–92.

56. Mandard AM, Dalibard F, Mandard JC, et al. Pathologic assessment of tumor regression after preoperative chemoradiotherapy of esophageal carcinoma. Clinicopathologic correlations. Cancer 1994;73(11):2680–6.

57. Korst RJ, Kansler AL, Port JL, et al. Downstaging of T or N predicts long-term survival after preoperative chemotherapy and radical resection for esophageal carcinoma. Ann Thorac Surg 2006;82(2):480–4 [discussion: 484–5].

58. Barbour AP, Jones M, Gonen M, et al. Refining esophageal cancer staging after neoadjuvant therapy: importance of treatment response. Ann Surg Oncol 2008;15(10):2894–902.

59. Geh JI, Bond SJ, Bentzen SM, et al. Systematic overview of preoperative (neoadjuvant) chemoradiotherapy trials in oesophageal cancer: evidence of a radiation and chemotherapy dose response. Radiother Oncol 2006;78(3):236–44.

60. Solomon N, Zhuge Y, Cheung M, et al. The roles of neoadjuvant radiotherapy and lymphadenectomy in the treatment of esophageal adenocarcinoma. Ann Surg Oncol 2010;17(3):791–803.

61. Mulligan ED, Dunne B, Griffin M, et al. Margin involvement and outcome in oesophageal carcinoma: a 10-year experience in a specialist unit. Eur J Surg Oncol 2004;30(3):313–7.

62. Sujendran V, Wheeler J, Baron R, et al. Effect of neoadjuvant chemotherapy on circumferential margin positivity and its impact on prognosis in patients with resectable oesophageal cancer. Br J Surg 2008;95(2):191–4.

63. Khan OA, Fitzgerald JJ, Soomro I, et al. Prognostic significance of circumferential resection margin involvement following oesophagectomy for cancer. Br J Cancer 2003;88(10):1549–52.

64. Kelly S, Harris KM, Berry E, et al. A systematic review of the staging performance of endoscopic ultrasound in gastro-oesophageal carcinoma. Gut 2001;49(4):534–9.

Adjuvant (Postoperative) Therapy for Esophageal Cancer

Geoffrey Y. Ku, MD, David H. Ilson, MD, PhD*

KEYWORDS

- Esophageal cancer • Gastroesophageal junction cancer • Adjuvant • Chemoradiation
- Chemotherapy

KEY POINTS

- In the past 10 to 15 years, completed clinical trials have demonstrated that some therapy in addition to surgery improves survival in patients with locally advanced cancers of the esophagus and gastroesophageal (GE) junction.
- In Europe and the United States, a common approach is to administer perioperative chemotherapy for resectable GE junction adenocarcinoma, based on the MAGIC study.
- Several trials, including the recent CROSS trial, also show a benefit for preoperative chemoradiation for tumors of the esophagus and GE junction.
- In Asia, recent trials in gastric adenocarcinoma have demonstrated a survival benefit for adjuvant chemotherapy, either with 1 year of the oral 5-fluorouracil prodrug S-1 or with 6 months of capecitabine/oxaliplatin therapy.
- A clearly proven strategy for squamous cell carcinomas is chemoradiation, administered either as preoperative therapy or as definitive treatment for patients who subsequently achieve a clinical complete response.

INTRODUCTION

In the United States, cancers of the esophagus and gastroesophageal (GE) junction are uncommon but aggressive. In 2013 an estimated 17,990 patients will be diagnosed, with an estimated 15,210 deaths from this disease.[1] These poor outcomes notwithstanding, survival has actually improved over time. In the period between 1975 to 1977 and 2000 to 2007, 5-year survival for esophageal cancers has increased from 5% to 19%.

Adenocarcinomas and squamous cell carcinomas (SCCs) account for 98% of all cases of esophageal cancer. SCCs normally occur in the upper two-thirds of the esophagus while adenocarcinomas occur in the lower third and at the GE junction. While cases of proximal esophageal SCCs have steadily declined (because of a parallel decrease in alcohol and tobacco consumption), the incidence of adenocarcinoma of the distal esophagus and GE junction has increased 4% to 10% per year among men in the United States since 1976.[2,3] Adenocarcinomas now account for more than 75% of esophageal tumors, and their increase is thought to be due to an increased incidence of gastroesophageal reflux disease[4] and obesity.[5]

In comparison to its relative rarity in the United States, esophageal cancer (predominantly SCC) is endemic in parts of East Asia, which account for more than half of the approximately 500,000 cases that develop per year (this number does not fully take into account GE junction tumors,

---

Disclosures: The authors have nothing to disclose.
Gastrointestinal Oncology Service, Department of Medicine, Memorial Sloan-Kettering Cancer Center, New York, NY 10065, USA
* Corresponding author. Memorial Sloan-Kettering Cancer Center, 300 East 66th Street, New York, NY 10065.
E-mail address: ilsond@mskcc.org

Thorac Surg Clin 23 (2013) 525–533
http://dx.doi.org/10.1016/j.thorsurg.2013.07.008

which may variously be categorized as gastric cancers).[6]

This review focuses specifically on adjuvant (postoperative) therapies for locally advanced esophageal and GE junction adenocarcinomas and SCCs (T3–4 or node-positive tumors), namely postoperative chemoradiation or chemotherapy. Where relevant, strategies that incorporate or consist of preoperative treatments are also discussed.

ADJUVANT CHEMORADIATION

In the United States, a standard of care is postoperative chemoradiation for resected GE junction adenocarcinomas, based primarily on the results of the Intergroup 116 trial.[7] This trial randomized 556 patients with gastric adenocarcinomas (20% of whom had tumors that involved the GE junction) to adjuvant chemotherapy and chemoradiation with bolus 5-fluorouracil (5-FU)/leucovorin versus observation alone following surgery. Patients who received adjuvant chemoradiation had an improvement in relapse-free survival (RFS) (3-year RFS 48% vs 31%, P<.001) and overall survival (OS) (3-year OS 51% vs 40%, P = .005). Despite these positive results, this trial is frequently criticized because of the relatively inadequate surgical resections that were performed: 54% of patients had less than a D1 or D2 resection, which is less than a complete dissection of the involved lymph nodes. It has been argued that radiation in this setting compensated for inadequate surgery because the greatest impact of adjuvant chemoradiation was a reduction in local recurrence of cancer. Such benefits may not be seen for radiotherapy if a more complete D1 or D2 surgical resection is undertaken. The size of the radiotherapy field for GE junction cancers, extending from the surgical bed high into the mediastinum to cover the anastomosis, is likely to exacerbate toxicity, and reinforces the application of preoperative rather than postoperative chemoradiation for these patients.

Based on the results of the Intergroup trial, the CALGB (Cancer and Leukemia Group B) 80101 trial attempted to intensify adjuvant chemoradiation by adding the ECF regimen (epirubicin/cisplatin/infusional 5-FU) as part of adjuvant treatment combined with 5-FU and radiation. Five hundred forty-six patients with gastric cancer (30% of whom had tumors involving the GE junction and proximal stomach) were enrolled. The standard arm consisted of systemic bolus 5-FU/leucovorin preceding and following chemoradiation with infusional 5-FU while the experimental arm intensified the systemic chemotherapy by replacing the bolus 5-FU/leucovorin with the ECF regimen. Results

were recently presented in abstract form, and reveal no improvement in 3-year disease-free survival (DFS; 47% vs 46%) or OS (52% vs 50%) with the addition of an anthracycline and platinum compound to 5-FU.[8] These results are also virtually identical to the outcomes in the adjuvant chemoradiation arm of the Intergroup 116 trial. These findings indicate that 5-FU monotherapy, combined with radiation, remains a standard of care, and that adding cisplatin and epirubicin to adjuvant chemotherapy failed to improve survival. ECF should not be used as an adjuvant chemotherapy regimen, although preoperative and postoperative ECF without radiation therapy remains a care standard (see later discussion).

The results of the aforementioned studies are summarized in **Table 1**.

ADJUVANT CHEMOTHERAPY

In comparison with chemoradiation, trials in East Asia of resectable gastric cancer have frequently focused on postoperative chemotherapy alone. To date, 2 large phase III trials have demonstrated a benefit for this approach. These data support the use of adjuvant fluoropyrimidines as monotherapy, and combination chemotherapy with a fluoropyrimidine plus a platinum agent. The results are summarized in **Table 2**, but should be interpreted with considerable caution because these trials have exclusively enrolled patients with gastric adenocarcinoma. In East Asia, less than 10% of tumors occur in the proximal stomach/GE junction, making it unclear whether they are applicable to the patient population discussed in this article.

The ACTS-GC (Adjuvant Chemotherapy Trial of TS-1 for Gastric Cancer) study was performed in Japan. In this study of 1059 patients with completely resected (R0) stage II/III gastric cancer who had undergone D2 resections, patients were randomized to 1 year of adjuvant S-1 versus observation.[9] S-1 is a mixture of tegafur (an oral 5-FU prodrug), gimeracil (a dihydropyrimidine dehydrogenase inhibitor that may potentiate the effect of 5-FU), and oteracil (which may reduce the gastrointestinal toxicity of 5-FU). Five-year outcomes for this trial were recently updated, confirming that adjuvant S-1 is associated with significant improvements in 5-year RFS (65.4% vs 53.1%, hazard ratio [HR] 0.65, 95% confidence interval [CI] 0.54–0.79) and OS (71.7% vs 61.1%, HR 0.67, 95% CI 0.54–0.83) compared with observation alone.[10] Subgroup analyses revealed benefit for all groups, including by stage and histologic type.

The second trial is the CLASSIC trial (capecitabine and oxaliplatin adjuvant study in stomach

Table 1
Results of phase III postoperative chemoradiation trials in gastric cancer and GE junction cancer

Treatment	Histology	No. of Patients	Disease-Free Survival		Overall Survival		Local Failure[a] (%)
			Median	Overall	Median	Overall	
Surgery	Adeno	275	**19 mo**	3-y **31%**	**27 mo**	3-y **41%**	29
Postop. 5-FU/LV → 5-FU/RT → 5-FU/LV		281	**30 mo**	3-y **48%**	**36 mo**	3-y **50%**	19
Postop. 5-FU/LV → 5-FU/RT → 5-FU/LV	Adeno	280	30 mo	3-y 46%	36.6 mo	3-y 50% 5-y 41%	NS
Postop. ECF → 5-FU/RT → ECF		266	28 mo	3-y 47%	37.8 mo	3-y 52% 5-y 44%	NS

Numbers in bold indicate statistically significant differences.
Abbreviations: Adeno, adenocarcinoma; ECF, epirubicin/cisplatin/infusional 5-fluorouracil; LV, leucovorin; NS, not stated; RT, radiotherapy.
[a] Local failure with or without distant recurrence.
Data from Macdonald JS, Smalley SR, Benedetti J, et al. Chemoradiotherapy after surgery compared with surgery alone for adenocarcinoma of the stomach or gastroesophageal junction. N Engl J Med 2001;345:725–30; and Fuchs C, Tepper J, Niedzwiecki D, et al. Postoperative adjuvant chemoradiation for gastric or gastroesophageal junction (GEJ) adenocarcinoma using epirubicin, cisplatin, and infusional (CI) 5-FU (ECF) before and after CI 5-FU and radiotherapy (CRT) compared with bolus 5-FU/LV before and after CRT: intergroup trial CALGB 80101 [abstract]. J Clin Oncol 2011;29:4003.

cancer), which was performed in 1035 East Asian patients who had undergone an R0, D2 resection of gastric cancer of stage II to IIIB.[11] Patients were randomized to 6 months of adjuvant capecitabine/oxaliplatin versus observation. While OS data remain immature, adjuvant chemotherapy was associated with an improvement in 3-year DFS (74% vs 59%, HR 0.56, 95% CI 0.44–0.72; P<.0001).

In comparison with these studies, 2 Japanese studies that evaluated adjuvant chemotherapy, with either cisplatin/vindesine[12] or 5-FU/cisplatin,[13] for resected esophageal SCCs reported no clear benefit. Whereas the trial with cisplatin/vindesine did not show any survival benefit, the trial with 5-FU/cisplatin did reveal an improvement in DFS but not OS, but only for patients with lymph node involvement (5-year DFS 52% vs 38%). Taken together, there are no clear data to suggest benefit for adjuvant chemotherapy in resected SCCs.

PERIOPERATIVE CHEMOTHERAPY

A strategy of perioperative chemotherapy is the predominant approach in Europe and also in the United States, based primarily on the phase III MAGIC (Medical Research Council Adjuvant Gastric Infusional Chemotherapy) trial performed in the United Kingdom.[14] This trial randomized 503 patients with gastric adenocarcinomas (26% of whom had tumors in the lower esophagus/GE junction) to 3 cycles each of preoperative and postoperative ECF and surgery, or surgery alone. Perioperative chemotherapy resulted in significant

improvement in 5-year OS (36% vs 23%, P = .009), establishing this regimen as a standard of care.

A similar degree of benefit was also noted in the contemporaneous French FFCD 9703 trial of 224 patients with esophagogastric adenocarcinoma (75% had tumors in the lower esophagus and GE junction).[15] Patients were randomized to 6 cycles of perioperative 5-FU/cisplatin followed by surgery versus surgery alone. Perioperative chemotherapy on this trial was associated with a significant improvement in 5-year DFS (34% vs 19%, P = .003) and OS (38% vs 24%, P = .02). Although comparisons between different clinical trials must be made cautiously, the survival benefit seen with 5-FU/cisplatin on this trial appears to be nearly identical to that seen with ECF in the MAGIC trial.

Aside from these 2 positive trials (which exclusively enrolled patients with adenocarcinoma histology), other phase III evaluations of preoperative or perioperative chemotherapy in esophageal cancers either have been negative or have had more marginal benefit. The North American Intergroup 113 trial failed to show a survival benefit for perioperative 5-FU/cisplatin in 440 patients with esophageal cancer (approximately half of whom had adenocarcinomas; eligibility limited extension of the tumor to 2 cm beyond the GE junction into the stomach).[16] The MRC OEO-2 trial, which randomized 802 patients to surgery alone versus 2 cycles of preoperative 5-FU/cisplatin, reported a modest improvement in 5-year OS with chemotherapy (23% vs 17%, P = .03).[17] Two-thirds of patients

Table 2
Results of phase III preoperative, perioperative, or postoperative chemotherapy trials in esophageal cancer and GE junction cancer

Treatment	Histology	No. of Patients	R0 Resection Rate (%)	Pathologic CR Rate (%)	Survival Median	Survival Overall	Local Failure[a] (%)
Periop. ECF + surgery	Adeno	250	69	0	**24 mo**	5-y **36%**	14
Surgery		253	66	N/A	**20 mo**	5-y **23%**	21
Periop. 5-FU/Cis + surgery	Adeno	109	**87**	NS	NS	5-y **38%**	24
Surgery		110	**74**	N/A	NS	5-y **24%**	26
Periop. 5-FU/Cis + surgery	Adeno (54%) +	213	62	2.5	14.9 mo	3-y 23%	32
Surgery	SCC	227	59	N/A	16.1 mo	3-y 26%	31
Preop. 5-FU/Cis + surgery	Adeno (66%) +	400	**60**	NS	**16.8 mo**	5-y 23%	19
Surgery	SCC	402	**54**	N/A	**13.3 mo**	5-y 17%	17
Preop. 5-FU/LV/Cis + surgery	Adeno	72	**82**	7.1	64.6 mo	2-y 73%	NS
Surgery		72	**67**	N/A	52.5 mo	2-y 70%	NS
Surgery	Adeno	530	N/A		NR	5-y **61%**	2.8
Surgery + S-1		529			NR	5-y **72%**	1.3
Surgery	Adeno	515	N/A		NR[b]	3-y[b] **59%**	44
Surgery + Capeox		520			NR[b]	3-y[b] **74%**	21
Surgery	SCC	100	N/A		NS	5-y 45%	23
Surgery + Cis/vindesine		105			NS	5-y 48%	21
Surgery	SCC	122	N/A		NS	5-y 52%	86
Surgery + 5-FU/Cis		120			NS	5-y 61%	80

Numbers in bold indicate statistically significant differences.

Abbreviations: 5-FU, 5-fluorouracil; Adeno, adenocarcinoma; bleo, bleomycin; Capeox, capecitabine/oxaliplatin; Cis, cisplatin; CR, complete response; ECF, epirubicin/cisplatin/5-fluoruoracil; N/A, not applicable; NR, not reached; NS, not stated; SCC, squamous cell carcinoma.

[a] Local failure with or without distant recurrence.

[b] Disease-free survival.

Data from Refs.[9–18,37]

had adenocarcinomas and three-quarters of tumors were in the lower esophagus or gastric cardia. The limited benefit in this trial was purportedly because of improvements in the R0 resection rate favoring the use of preoperative chemotherapy, with no impact of chemotherapy on distant recurrence. This observation is also at odds with the Intergroup 113 trial which, in addition to failing to improve survival, failed to improve rates of R0 resection when preoperative chemotherapy was administered. Most recently, the European EORTC 40954 trial evaluated a strategy of preoperative 5-FU/leucovorin/cisplatin in 144 patients with GE junction and gastric adenocarcinoma.[18] The trial was stopped because of poor accrual, which limits the power of the study, and no differences in survival were detected. An improvement in the R0 resection rate in the preoperative chemotherapy group in this trial failed to translate into any survival benefit.

These data are summarized in **Table 2**. An updated meta-analysis by Sjoquist and colleagues[19] of 10 randomized trials involving preoperative chemotherapy for esophageal and GE junction cancers suggested a 13% decreased risk of all-cause mortality for this approach in patients with adenocarcinomas versus surgery alone (HR 0.87, 95% CI 0.79–0.96; P<.005). In this meta-analysis, both the MAGIC and EORTC 40954 trials were excluded because outcomes were not stratified based on gastric versus GE junction tumors.

By comparison, evidence of benefit for preoperative chemotherapy in SCC histology is very limited. Preoperative chemotherapy based on the MRC OEO-2 trial is theoretically an option, but only about one-third of the patients on this trial had SCC histology, and the 6% improvement in survival outcomes with preoperative chemotherapy for the overall intention-to-treat population is relatively modest. This small benefit must also be weighed against the lack of improvement noted in the Intergroup 113 trial, the other trial that also treated SCC patients. Not surprisingly, the meta-analysis by Sjoquist and colleagues[19] does not show a clear improvement in survival for preoperative chemotherapy in patients with SCC (HR 0.92, 95% CI 0.81–1.04; $P = .18$).

PREOPERATIVE CHEMORADIATION

While there are proven postoperative strategies that improve outcomes for resected esophageal adenocarcinomas (as discussed above), no such data exist for resected SCCs. Instead, validated approaches for SCCs include preoperative chemoradiation. Six contemporary randomized trials have compared preoperative chemoradiation followed by surgery versus surgery alone for esophageal and GE junction tumors (both adenocarcinomas and SCCs).[20–25] Of these, 3 have been positive and have revealed a survival benefit for this approach. These results are summarized in **Table 3**.

Overall, many of the randomized trials are associated with methodological concerns (including the lack of rigorous pretherapy staging with endoscopic ultrasonography and/or laparoscopy) and are significantly smaller than randomized preoperative chemotherapy trials (eg, the positive CALGB 9781 study enrolled only 56 patients). Although the results of these trials are conflicting, they do at a minimum suggest improved curative resection rates as well as decreased local recurrence.

A potential new standard of care was established by the rigorously conducted Dutch CROSS trial.[24] In this study of 366 evaluable patients with esophageal tumors (of which 75% and 65%, respectively, were adenocarcinomas and lymph node positive by endoscopic ultrasonography), patients were randomized to preoperative carboplatin/paclitaxel combined with 41.4 Gy of

Table 3
Results of phase III preoperative chemoradiation trials in esophageal cancer and GE junction cancer

Treatment	Histology	No. of Patients	R0 Resection Rate (%)	Pathologic CR Rate (%)	Survival Median	Survival Overall	Local Failure (%)	Reference
Preop. CRT	Adeno	50	45	24	16.9 mo	3-y 30%	19	Urba et al,[23] 2001
Surgery	(76%) + SCC	50	45	N/A	17.6 mo	3-y 16%	42	
Preop. CRT	Adeno	58	NS	25	**16 mo**	3-y **32%**	NS	Walsh et al,[25] 1996
Surgery		55		N/A	**11 mo**	3-y **6%**		
Preop. CRT	SCC	143	81	26	18.6 mo	5-y 26%	NS	Bosset et al,[20] 1997
Surgery		139	69	N/A	18.6 mo	5-y 26%		
Preop. CRT	Adeno	128	**80**	9	22.2 mo	NS	15	Burmeister et al,[21] 2005
Surgery	(63%) + SCC + other	128	59	N/A	19.3 mo	NS	26	
Preop. CRT	Adeno	30	NS	40	**4.5 y**	5-y **39%**	NS	Tepper et al,[22] 2008
Surgery	(75%) + SCC	26		N/A	**1.8 y**	5-y **16%**		
Preop. CRT	Adeno	178	**92**	29	**49.4 mo**	3-y **58%**	NS	van Hagen et al,[24] 2012
Surgery	(74%) + SCC	188	69	N/A	**24.0 mo**	3-y **44%**		

Numbers in bold indicate statistically significant differences.

Abbreviations: Adeno, adenocarcinoma; CR, complete response; N/A, not applicable; NS, not stated; Preop. CRT, preoperative chemoradiation; SCC, squamous cell carcinoma.

Data from Refs.[20–25]

radiation versus surgery alone. Preoperative chemoradiation resulted in an improvement in R0 resection rates (92% vs 67%, P<.001), in a pathologic complete response (pCR) rate of 29% (23% for adenocarcinoma and 49% for SCC), and in improved OS compared with surgery alone (median OS 49.4 vs 24.0 months, 3-year OS 58% vs 44%; P = .003). Preoperative therapy was also relatively well tolerated, with mostly grade 3 toxicities noted in only 20% of patients (13% nonhematologic, 7% hematologic). There did appear to be a greater degree of benefit for patients with SCC versus adenocarcinoma histology (univariate HR for death 0.45 vs 0.73), but all patients derived benefit. Although this study demonstrates a clear benefit for chemoradiation, it is not possible to definitively conclude that carboplatin/paclitaxel is the preferred regimen combined with radiation relative to standard fluoropyrimidine/platinum doublet used in other trials. Nevertheless, the pCR rate of 49% in SCC is the highest ever reported in a phase III trial, while the pCR rate of 23% for adenocarcinomas compares favorably with other phase II/III studies. Coupled with the ease of administration and tolerability, carboplatin/paclitaxel may be considered the new standard of care and the reference regimen for future trial design.

A benefit for preoperative chemoradiation is supported by the previously discussed meta-analysis in which 13 randomized trials of preoperative chemoradiation (including the 5 trials discussed above) were analyzed.[19] Preoperative chemoradiation was associated with a decreased risk of all-cause mortality of 25% (HR 0.75, 95% CI 0.59–0.95; P = .02) in patients with adenocarcinoma histology versus surgery alone. A similar degree of benefit was seen in SCC patients (HR 0.80, 95% CI 0.68–0.93; P = .004).

PREOPERATIVE VERSUS DEFINITIVE CHEMORADIATION FOR SCC

Two randomized trials have compared definitive chemoradiation with chemoradiation followed by surgery. The first study was performed by the German Esophageal Cancer Study Group, which assigned 172 patients with SCC to preoperative therapy (3 cycles of cisplatin/5-FU/leucovorin/etoposide, then cisplatin/etoposide and concurrent radiation to 40 Gy) followed by surgery or to the preoperative therapy alone with a higher radiation dose (to at least 65 Gy) in lieu of surgery.[26] Although local progression-free survival was improved with the addition of surgery (HR for chemoradiation-only group vs surgery group 2.1, 95% CI 1.3–3.5; P = .003), there was only

a nonsignificant trend toward improvement in 3-year OS (31.3% vs 24.4%). Treatment-related mortality was also significantly higher in the surgery group than in the chemoradiation-only group (12.8% vs 3.5%). Ten-year survival data for this trial were recently presented in abstract form, reaffirming the absence of a significant difference between both groups.[27]

The second study is the French FFCD 9102 trial, in which 444 eligible patients with mostly SCC histology underwent initial chemoradiation with cisplatin/5-FU.[28] Those who demonstrated a response to initial therapy were then randomized to either undergo surgery or receive an additional 3 cycles of cisplatin/5-FU with radiation, as the investigators considered that it would be inappropriate to continue chemoradiation in patients not responding to therapy. Of the 444 patients, 259 were randomized. The 2-year survival rate was not significantly different between both groups (34% in the surgery group vs 40% in the chemoradiation-only group; P = .44). However, locoregional recurrence was higher in the chemoradiation-only group (43% vs 34%) and there was also a higher incidence of stent placement in this group (32% vs 5%). Three-month mortality was significantly higher in the surgery group (9.3% vs 0.8%). Based on these data, the investigators concluded that patients with tumors, especially of SCC histology, who responded to initial chemoradiation did not derive any survival benefit from subsequent surgery. Patients who underwent surgery did have improved local control of their disease, albeit at the cost of increased treatment-related mortality.

An interesting question that arises from this study is whether patients who do not respond to initial therapy benefit from subsequent surgery. In an abstract, Jouve and colleagues[29] discussed the outcome of the 192 of the 451 registered patients from the aforementioned FFCD study who were not randomized to further protocol therapy after initial chemotherapy, primarily because of a lack of response but also because of medical contraindication or patient refusal. Of these nonrandomized patients, 112 subsequently underwent surgery, with 80 undergoing R0 resections. The median OS for the patients who underwent surgery was significantly superior to the median OS of those who did not (17.3 vs 6.1 months), and was comparable with the median OS of the patients who were randomized. Although there are clear limitations and potential strong confounders to such an analysis, these data may suggest that salvage esophagectomy can be beneficial for a subset of patients who do not respond to initial therapy. A constant and important consideration is the high rate of development of metastatic disease within the first 2 years of diagnosis, a rate exceeding 50% to 60% despite chemoradiation and surgery, which makes the selective application of surgery more of a justifiable approach in appropriate patients.

TARGETED THERAPIES

As with many other solid tumor malignancies, targeted therapies have also been the subject of intense interest. While many ongoing trials are evaluating exclusively preoperative strategies, the United Kingdom MAGIC-B trial (NCT00450203) is randomizing patients with locally advanced GE junction and gastric cancer to perioperative ECX chemotherapy (epirubicin/cisplatin/capecitabine) with or without bevacizumab, a monoclonal antibody against vascular endothelial growth factor. However, 2 phase II trials combining bevacizumab (alone[30] or with erlotinib,[31] an oral tyrosine kinase inhibitor against epidermal growth factor receptor [EGFR]) with preoperative chemoradiation have failed to show an improvement in outcomes in comparison with historical controls. The phase III AVAGAST trial, which added bevacizumab to chemotherapy for advanced gastric cancer, also failed to meet its primary end point of improving OS.[32]

In addition, phase III evaluations of agents that target the EGFR (cetuximab,[33] panitumumab,[34] and erlotinib[35]) in the metastatic setting or in the locally advanced setting (combined with chemoradiation)[36] have been disappointing. These trials have suggested either no benefit or deleterious effects with the addition of these targeted agents to standard therapy.

SUMMARY

In the past 10 to 15 years, completed clinical trials have clearly demonstrated that some therapy in addition to surgery improves survival in patients with locally advanced esophageal and GE junction cancers. These trials have not established an optimal strategy, but several postoperative and perioperative approaches, which all result in absolute improvements in survival of approximately 15% over surgery alone but have not been compared head to head, are validated.

In Europe and the United States, a common approach is to administer perioperative chemotherapy for resectable GE junction adenocarcinoma, based on the MAGIC study. For patients who undergo upfront surgery for a GE junction adenocarcinoma, the United States Intergroup 116 trial also demonstrated improved survival,

but it is frequently argued that radiation was compensating for suboptimal surgery in this study. Several trials, including the recent CROSS trial, also show a benefit of preoperative chemoradiation for esophageal and GE junction tumors.

In Asia, where patients typically undergo upfront D2 gastrectomies, recent trials in gastric adenocarcinoma have demonstrated a survival benefit for adjuvant chemotherapy, either with 1 year of the oral 5-FU prodrug S-1 or with 6 months of capecitabine/oxaliplatin. Whether such a benefit for adjuvant chemotherapy alone exists for GE junction adenocarcinomas is not clear because most of these trials enrolled patients with distal gastric cancer.

All of these postoperative approaches apply only to adenocarcinomas. A clearly proven strategy for SCCs is chemoradiation, administered either as preoperative therapy or as definitive treatment for patients who subsequently achieve a clinical complete response. A small benefit has also been shown for preoperative chemotherapy for SCC tumors in 1 of 2 phase III trials.

REFERENCES

1. Siegel R, Naishadham D, Jemal A. Cancer statistics. CA Cancer J Clin 2013;63:11–30.
2. Crew KD, Neugut AI. Epidemiology of upper gastrointestinal malignancies. Semin Oncol 2004;31: 450–64.
3. Devesa SS, Fraumeni JF Jr. The rising incidence of gastric cardia cancer. J Natl Cancer Inst 1999;91: 747–9.
4. Rubenstein JH, Taylor JB. Meta-analysis: the association of oesophageal adenocarcinoma with symptoms of gastro-oesophageal reflux. Aliment Pharmacol Ther 2010;32:1222–7.
5. Hampel H, Abraham NS, El-Serag HB. Meta-analysis: obesity and the risk for gastroesophageal reflux disease and its complications. Ann Intern Med 2005;143:199–211.
6. Ferlay J, Shin HR, Bray F, et al. Estimates of worldwide burden of cancer in 2008: GLOBOCAN 2008. Int J Cancer 2010;127:2893–917.
7. Macdonald JS, Smalley SR, Benedetti J, et al. Chemoradiotherapy after surgery compared with surgery alone for adenocarcinoma of the stomach or gastroesophageal junction. N Engl J Med 2001; 345:725–30.
8. Fuchs C, Tepper J, Niedzwiecki D, et al. Postoperative adjuvant chemoradiation for gastric or gastroesophageal junction (GEJ) adenocarcinoma using epirubicin, cisplatin, and infusional (CI) 5-FU (ECF) before and after CI 5-FU and radiotherapy (CRT) compared with bolus 5-FU/LV before and after

CRT: Intergroup trial CALGB 80101 [abstract]. J Clin Oncol 2011;29:4003.

9. Sakuramoto S, Sasako M, Yamaguchi T, et al. Adjuvant chemotherapy for gastric cancer with S-1, an oral fluoropyrimidine. N Engl J Med 2007;357:1810–20.

10. Sasako M, Sakuramoto S, Katai H, et al. Five-year outcomes of a randomized phase III trial comparing adjuvant chemotherapy with S-1 versus surgery alone in stage II or III gastric cancer. J Clin Oncol 2011;29:4387–93.

11. Bang YJ, Kim YW, Yang HK, et al. Adjuvant capecitabine and oxaliplatin for gastric cancer after D2 gastrectomy (CLASSIC): a phase 3 open-label, randomised controlled trial. Lancet 2012;379:315–21.

12. Ando N, Iizuka T, Kakegawa T, et al. A randomized trial of surgery with and without chemotherapy for localized squamous carcinoma of the thoracic esophagus: the Japan Clinical Oncology Group Study. J Thorac Cardiovasc Surg 1997;114:205–9.

13. Ando N, Iizuka T, Ide H, et al. Surgery plus chemotherapy compared with surgery alone for localized squamous cell carcinoma of the thoracic esophagus: a Japan Clinical Oncology Group Study—JCOG9204. J Clin Oncol 2003;21:4592–6.

14. Cunningham D, Allum WH, Stenning SP, et al. Perioperative chemotherapy versus surgery alone for resectable gastroesophageal cancer. N Engl J Med 2006;355:11–20.

15. Ychou M, Boige V, Pignon JP, et al. Perioperative chemotherapy compared with surgery alone for resectable gastroesophageal adenocarcinoma: an FNCLCC and FFCD multicenter phase III trial. J Clin Oncol 2011;29:1715–21.

16. Kelsen DP, Ginsberg R, Pajak TF, et al. Chemotherapy followed by surgery compared with surgery alone for localized esophageal cancer. N Engl J Med 1998;339:1979–84.

17. Allum WH, Stenning SP, Bancewicz J, et al. Long-term results of a randomized trial of surgery with or without preoperative chemotherapy in esophageal cancer. J Clin Oncol 2009;27:5062–7.

18. Schuhmacher C, Gretschel S, Lordick F, et al. Neoadjuvant chemotherapy compared with surgery alone for locally advanced cancer of the stomach and cardia: European Organisation for Research and Treatment of Cancer randomized trial 40954. J Clin Oncol 2010;28:5210–8.

19. Sjoquist KM, Burmeister BH, Smithers BM, et al. Survival after neoadjuvant chemotherapy or chemoradiotherapy for resectable oesophageal carcinoma: an updated meta-analysis. Lancet Oncol 2011;12:681–92.

20. Bosset JF, Gignoux M, Triboulet JP, et al. Chemoradiotherapy followed by surgery compared with surgery alone in squamous-cell cancer of the esophagus. N Engl J Med 1997;337:161–7.

21. Burmeister BH, Smithers BM, Gebski V, et al. Surgery alone versus chemoradiotherapy followed by surgery for resectable cancer of the oesophagus: a randomised controlled phase III trial. Lancet Oncol 2005;6:659–68.

22. Tepper J, Krasna MJ, Niedzwiecki D, et al. Phase III trial of trimodality therapy with cisplatin, fluorouracil, radiotherapy, and surgery compared with surgery alone for esophageal cancer: CALGB 9781. J Clin Oncol 2008;26:1086–92.

23. Urba SG, Orringer MB, Turrisi A, et al. Randomized trial of preoperative chemoradiation versus surgery alone in patients with locoregional esophageal carcinoma. J Clin Oncol 2001;19:305–13.

24. van Hagen P, Hulshof MC, van Lanschot JJ, et al. Preoperative chemoradiotherapy for esophageal or junctional cancer. N Engl J Med 2012;366:2074–84.

25. Walsh TN, Noonan N, Hollywood D, et al. A comparison of multimodal therapy and surgery for esophageal adenocarcinoma. N Engl J Med 1996;335:462–7.

26. Stahl M, Stuschke M, Lehmann N, et al. Chemoradiation with and without surgery in patients with locally advanced squamous cell carcinoma of the esophagus. J Clin Oncol 2005;23:2310–7.

27. Stahl M, Wilke H, Lehmann N, et al, Group GOCS. Long-term results of a phase III study investigating chemoradiation with and without surgery in locally advanced squamous cell carcinoma (LA-SCC) of the esophagus [abstract]. J Clin Oncol 2008;26:4530.

28. Bedenne L, Michel P, Bouche O, et al. Chemoradiation followed by surgery compared with chemoradiation alone in squamous cancer of the esophagus: FFCD 9102. J Clin Oncol 2007;25:1160–8.

29. Jouve J, Michel P, Mariette C, et al. Outcome of the nonrandomized patients in the FFCD 9102 trial: chemoradiation followed by surgery compared with chemoradiation alone in squamous cancer of the esophagus [abstract]. J Clin Oncol 2008;26:4555.

30. Ilson D, Goodman K, Janjigian Y, et al. Phase II trial of bevacizumab, irinotecan, cisplatin, and radiation as preoperative therapy in esophageal adenocarcinoma [abstract]. J Clin Oncol 2012;30:67.

31. Bendell JC, Meluch A, Peyton J, et al. A phase II trial of preoperative concurrent chemotherapy/radiation therapy plus bevacizumab/erlotinib in the treatment of localized esophageal cancer. Clin Adv Hematol Oncol 2012;10:430–7.

32. Ohtsu A, Shah MA, Van Cutsem E, et al. Bevacizumab in combination with chemotherapy as first-line therapy in advanced gastric cancer: a randomized, double-blind, placebo-controlled phase III study. J Clin Oncol 2011;29:3968–76.

33. Lordick F, Bodoky G, Chung H, et al. Cetuximab in combination with capecitabine and cisplatin as first-line treatment in advanced gastric cancer:

randomized controlled phase III EXPAND study [abstract]. Ann Oncol 2012;23:LBA3.

34. Waddell T, Chau I, Barbachano Y, et al. A randomized multicenter trial of epirubicin, oxaliplatin, and capecitabine (EOC) plus panitumumab in advanced esophagogastric cancer (REAL3) [abstract]. J Clin Oncol 2012;30:LBA4000.

35. Ferry D, Dutton S, Mansoor W, et al. Phase III multi-centre, randomised, double-blind, placebo-controlled trial of gefitinib versus placebo in esophageal cancer progressing after chemotherapy, COG (Cancer Oesophagus Gefitinib) [abstract]. Ann Oncol 2012;23:LBA20.

36. Crosby T, Hurt C, Falk S, et al. SCOPE 1: a phase II/III trial of chemoradiotherapy in esophageal cancer plus or minus cetuximab [abstract]. J Clin Oncol 2013;30:LBA3.

37. Medical Research Council Oesophageal Cancer Working Group. Surgical resection with or without preoperative chemotherapy in oesophageal cancer: a randomised controlled trial. Lancet 2002;359: 1727–33.

Update on Clinical Impact, Documentation, and Management of Complications Associated with Esophagectomy

Donald E. Low, FRCS(C)*, Artur Bodnar, MD

KEYWORDS

- Esophageal cancer • Complications • Esophagectomy • Clavien • Accordion
- Standardized pathways

KEY POINTS

- Complications associated with esophagectomy impact mortality, quality of life, costs, and survival.
- There is currently no standardized system for documenting postesophagectomy complications, which impedes comparisons of outcomes and quality improvement programs.
- The Accordion and Clavien systems are internationally recognized approaches to assessing complication severity and resource utilization and should be a component of all institutional and national databases.
- New endoscopic and interventional approaches to treating anastomotic leak and stricture and chyle leak can selectively decrease length of stay and costs of managing these complications.

EFFECT OF COMPLICATIONS ON OUTCOMES OF ESOPHAGEAL RESECTION FOR CANCER

The incidence of esophageal cancer continues to increase, especially in men. Surgery has historically been a major component of the treatment of nonmetastatic esophageal cancer, but its role is being reassessed in patients with high-grade dysplasia and superficial (T1a) cancer, and in patients with squamous cell carcinoma. With respect to mortality, esophagectomy remains an outlier compared with other major cancer procedures, which is highlighted in a review of Medicare patients up to 2008. This review demonstrated that although overall mortality rates are decreasing, mortality in the United States in patients older than 65 remained at 9%, 30% higher than any other major cancer operation.[1]

Mortality has long been linked to the volume of resections done by individual surgeons and medical centers. A recent meta-analysis of this relationship has confirmed a threefold increase in mortality in low-volume versus high-volume centers.[2] It is increasingly apparent, however, that mortality, along with other important outcome measures, can be improved in high-volume centers, but that the volume of esophageal resections

Disclosures: The authors have nothing to disclose.
Department of Thoracic Surgery and Thoracic Oncology, Virginia Mason Medical Center, 1100 Ninth Avenue, Seattle, WA 98111, USA
* Corresponding author. Section of General Thoracic Surgery, Virginia Mason Medical Center, 1100 Ninth Avenue, C6-SUR, Seattle, WA 98111.
E-mail address: gtsdel@vmmc.org

is a surrogate for many other issues, including specialized thoracic anesthesia and interventional gastroenterology and radiology departments, dedicated intensive care units (ICUs), as well as the application of standardized pathways and improved patient communication typically associated with oncologic nurse coordinators. A report reviewing the results from the Society of Thoracic Surgeons (STS) database did not demonstrate a direct association with high-volume centers and morbidity and mortality.[3] This may be due to the observation that high-volume surgeons are more likely to be located in academic institutions and have cardiothoracic training.[4]

In addition, the definition for "high volume" continues to be elusive. The Leapfrog Group, an independent organization monitoring risk-adjusted mortality, identified 13 per year as high volume.[5] Other reports use 20 per year as high volume,[6] whereas a report from the Dutch National Medical Registry sets the bar at 50 per year as high volume.[7]

There is currently no generally accepted system for categorizing, either the occurrence or severity of complications associated with esophageal resection. This has led to significant difficulty in comparing results both nationally and internationally, and in consistently documenting the true incidence of complications in individual reports and national audits. A recent report comparing outcomes in open versus minimally invasive esophageal resection highlighted the fact that overall morbidity was reported in only approximately 50% of publications and complication rates varied between 17% and 50%.[8] However, a report culminating in 2001 reviewing outcomes in Department of Veterans Affairs' medical centers in the United States, identified an overall complication rate of 49.5% at that time.[9]

There is evolving evidence that complications affect most major outcome measures with respect to the surgical treatment of esophageal cancer. The occurrence of intraoperative and postoperative complications have been directly linked to mortality,[10–12] length of stay,[11,13,14] and postoperative quality of life.[15–17] There is also evolving evidence demonstrating that complications affect the overall costs and resource utilization in major cancer surgery in general[18] and esophagectomy specifically.[13] There has been increasing assessment as to whether complications can affect survival after the treatment of esophageal cancer. There is evidence that complications affect the timing and incidence of cancer recurrence[19] and also affect long-term survival.[11,20] There is less evidence, however, that complications directly affect disease-free survival.[14,21]

What is clear is that complications are a major influence on both clinical and economic outcomes of esophageal resection, and methodologies to better categorize complications are essential for ongoing efforts to minimize their occurrence and impact.

CURRENT SYSTEMS FOR DOCUMENTING MORBIDITY ASSOCIATED WITH ESOPHAGECTOMY

Current assessment of complications lacks both consistency and standardization. An initial effort to assess the measurement and monitoring of surgical adverse events in 2001 reviewed 107 studies reporting outcomes in gastrointestinal surgery. They highlighted the fact that there were 40 different definitions of what constituted an anastomotic leak. Similarly, 82 studies described 41 definitions and 13 grading scales for surgical wound infection.[22]

A more recent systematic review of outcomes associated with esophagectomy reviewed 122 studies and reported that no single complication was reported in all articles and more than 60% of studies had no definitions for individual complications. Anastomotic leak rates were most commonly cited in 80% of articles but were defined in only 30% of reports with 22 different definitions. Blencowe and colleagues[10] concluded that "outcome reporting after esophageal cancer surgery is heterogeneous and inconsistent and lacks methodological rigor." They recommended the development of a consensus approach to reporting outcomes.

The lack of standardization and generally accepted definitions has been the case historically in open operations and confirmed more recently in a systematic review of minimally invasive esophagectomy.[23] The accuracy of reporting complications not only suffers from the lack of definitions of complications, but also from the lack of a generally accepted "statute of limitations" of when adverse events should be related to the surgical procedure. NSQIP recommends reporting complications up to 30 days following surgery. There is also no general consensus on a standard for reporting operative mortality associated with esophageal resection. However, a recent meta-analysis demonstrated that, if only 30-day mortality is reported, it would underestimate the postoperative mortality as manifested by in-hospital mortality by a factor of 4.[2]

A review of esophagectomy outcomes from 164 NSQIP hospitals demonstrated that even following case mix adjustment, results between institutions varied 161% for 30-day mortality and 84% for serious morbidity.[24] Some of this variation is a reflection of differences in service delivery, but equally it reflects the reality of the absence of a standardized reporting system for complications.

NEW SYSTEMS FOR STRATIFYING SEVERITY AND RESOURCE UTILIZATION OF COMPLICATIONS

There is general agreement that documentation of morbidity in most surgical procedures, but particularly esophagectomy, is done poorly because of the absence of a standardized system of definitions. Historically, complications have been recorded as individual occurrences or events. The identification and documentation of a complication is typically done by a wide variety of individuals, including surgeons, trainees, cancer coordinators, or data managers who have a variable degree of experience and clinical acumen. Recent assessments have indicated that the problem of consistency and classification of complications may reside in the recording physician.[25] Ideally, recording of complications should be done at several levels, using a consistent group of caregivers and in conjunction with independent data managers. The accuracy of the data will be improved with standardized definitions linked to an integrated method for assessing the severity of the complication, while at the same time recording the resources needed to deal with its occurrence.

Respiratory complications in general and pneumonia in particular are considered critically important adverse events with respect to esophagectomy outcomes (see "Respiratory Complications"). The vast majority of databases record pneumonia as an individual event. In fact, pneumonia can take the form of pulmonary infiltrates and fever, which can be treated with physical therapy or antibiotics. On the other hand, pneumonia can lead to hypoxia, necessitating a change in level of care or require bronchoscopy or minitracheostomy to manage pulmonary secretions. Pneumonia may also manifest as increasing pleural effusions that require additional surgical or radiologic drainage or even surgical intervention for empyema or trapped lung. Pneumonia can also continue to evolve to produce respiratory failure, requiring mechanical ventilation or tracheostomy. This example highlights the broad spectrum of severity and clinical response that cannot be adequately documented in a database with a data point: Pneumonia Yes/No.

It has been previously shown that the utility of a complication as a measure of quality depends on the magnitude of the problem measured in terms of both its incidence and its consequences.[26] Internationally, there are 2 current systems for grading complication severity and providing basic information on resource utilization. The Clavien system[27] is the most commonly applied system internationally, whereas the Accordion system is seeing increasing application in the United States.[28] The 2 classification systems are shown in **Table 1** and demonstrate significant similarities: grade I interventions typically involving bedside interventions; grade II involving predominately treatment modifications with drugs, transfusion, or nutrition; the higher grades documenting interventions either with or without general anesthesia; the highest grades involving single-organ or multiorgan failure; and ultimately the final grade documenting a complication resulting in death. Both systems have been validated as applicable and valuable in large series of esophageal resections[13,19] and other studies have demonstrated that Accordion or Clavien classification can be done retrospectively, seeing as the therapeutic interventions associated with complications are typically well documented in the chart or computerized record.[29] International trials such as the ROBOT trial, a randomized control trial assessing the difference in outcomes of robotically assisted, minimally invasive esophagectomy versus open transthoracic esophagectomy, have, as one of their primary outcome treatment assessments, the percentage of overall complications grade II or higher as rated by the Clavien system.[30] The importance and potential utility of these systems is further demonstrated by studies establishing a direct link between Accordion classification and length of stay and costs in the surgical management of esophageal cancer.[13]

A wide variety of vehicles have been used for the prediction and recording of outcomes, including complications in surgical procedures. The ASA (American Society of Anesthesia) score is the most commonly applied risk stratification system but is subjective and shows significant variation in how it is applied. Other systems for risk stratification, including Physiological and Operative Severity Score for the enUmeration of Mortality and morbidity (POSSUM) (Oesophageal-POSSUM),[31] surgical Apgar score,[32] Estimation of Physiologic Ability and Surgical Stress (EPASS),[33] and the National Cancer Institute Common Toxicity Criteria,[34] have all seen selective application. Although these systems have individual advantages, they have either not been validated or have seen limited international application.

Grotenhuis and colleagues[35] published experience with an individual nomogram from the 2 major

Table 1		
Dindo-Clavien or Accordion		
	Dindo-Clavien Classification of Surgical Complications	**Accordion Severity Classification of Postoperative Complications: Expanded Classification**
Grade I	Any deviation from the normal postoperative course without the need for pharmacologic treatment or surgical, endoscopic, and radiological interventions. Allowed therapeutic regimens are drugs as antiemetics, antipyretics, analgesics, diuretics, electrolytes, and physiotherapy. This grade also includes wound infections opened at the bedside.	1. *Mild Complication:* Requires only minor invasive procedures that can be done at the bedside, such as insertion of intravenous lines, urinary catheters, and nasogastric tubes, and drainage of wound infections. Physiotherapy and the following drugs are allowed: antiemetics, antipyretics, analgesics, diuretics, electrolytes, and physiotherapy.
Grade II	Requiring pharmacologic treatment with drugs other than such allowed for grade I complications. Blood transfusions and total parenteral nutrition are also included.	2. *Moderate Complication:* Requires pharmacologic treatment with drugs other than such allowed for minor complications, for instance antibiotics. Blood transfusions and total parenteral nutrition are also included.
Grade III	Requiring surgical, endoscopic, or radiological intervention.	
Grade IIIa	Intervention not under general anesthesia.	3. *Severe:* Invasive procedure without general anesthesia. Requires management by an endoscopic, interventional procedure or reoperation[a] without general anesthesia.
Grade IIIb	Intervention under general anesthesia.	4. *Severe:* Operation under general anesthesia. Requires management by an operation under general anesthesia.
Grade IV	Life-threatening complication (including CNS complications)[b] requiring IC/ICU management.	5. *Severe:* Organ system failure.[c]
Grade IVa	Single-organ dysfunction (including dialysis).	
Grade IVb	Multiorgan dysfunction.	
Grade V	Death of a patient.	6. *Death:* Postoperative death.
Suffix "d"	If the patient suffers from a complication at the time of discharge, the suffix "d" (for "disability") is added to the respective grade of complication. This label indicates the need for a follow-up to fully evaluate the complication.	

Abbreviations: CNS, central nervous system; IC, intermediate care; ICU, intensive care unit.
[a] An example would be a wound reexploration under conscious sedation and/or local anesthetic.
[b] Brain hemorrhage, ischemic stroke, and subarachnoidal bleeding, but excluding transient ischemic attacks.
[c] Such complications would normally be managed in an increased acuity setting but in some cases patients with complications of lower severity might also be admitted to an ICU.

cancer centers in the Netherlands attempting to predict the occurrence and severity of postoperative complications associated with esophagectomy. This system examined patient demographic and physiologic issues and used certain physiologic cardiopulmonary measures as well as an assessment of the proposed operative approach to assign a risk score. The system was found to be somewhat useful in the comparison between the 2 hospitals; however, the investigators summarized "that pre-operative prediction of complications in individual patients remains difficult, most likely due to the complexity of mechanisms causing these complications."

The current reality is that there is no standardized process for documenting complications after esophageal resection. However, the Clavien and Accordion systems provide an increasingly well-recognized international system for stratifying the severity of postoperative complications and documenting the resources that were required to treat individual complications. One of the limitations of both systems is that they classify only the most severe complication. Other methodologies are required to assess the severity and resource utilization in cases of multiple complications.

INFLUENCE OF OPERATIVE TECHNIQUE ON COMPLICATIONS

As the technical options for esophagectomy have evolved, the debate between surgeons as to the clinical and oncologic advantages of various surgical approaches has become more complex. Initial comparisons between open approaches highlighted the fact that the transhiatal operation was associated with an increased incidence of anastomotic and vocal cord complications, although the open transthoracic approach was generally recognized to have a higher instance of pulmonary and wound complications. A randomized trial from Germany in 2002 demonstrated that complications and costs of treatment were higher in transthoracic procedures, although mortality was seen to be equal.[36] There was a trend toward an improved 5-year survivorship in the transthoracic group, which did not reach statistical significance.[37] However, a subanalysis assessing the effect of tumor location (esophageal vs esophagogastric tumors) demonstrated a 14% survival advantage of esophageal tumors with a transthoracic approach.[38] Connors and colleagues[39] in 2007 carried out a comparison between open transhiatal and transthoracic esophagectomy, assessing 17,395 patients from the National In-Patient Sample. This article confirmed that high-volume hospitals overall provided better outcomes but there was no statistically significant difference in either mortality or morbidity between the 2 open operative approaches. Similar results were found in a study analyzing the Department of Veterans Affairs' National Surgical Quality Improvement Program involving 945 patients operated on over a 10-year period.[40]

The past 10 years has seen the increasing use of a variety of hybrid and exclusively minimally invasive operative approaches introduced to improve morbidity and mortality. Published indications from specialty surveys and national audits would indicate that currently between 14% and 31% of operations are done using minimally invasive techniques.[41,42] There have been multiple uncontrolled retrospective assessments comparing minimally invasive and open operative procedures. These assessments infer that minimally invasive operations typically take longer but are associated with less blood loss. There are also increasing indications that minimally invasive approaches can be associated with a lower incidence of respiratory complications.[43,44]

A recent randomized controlled trial from Europe assessed outcomes with open versus minimally invasive approaches. The trial did not demonstrate any difference in mortality but indicated that minimally invasive approaches had a lower incidence of pulmonary infections and better short-term quality of life. However, the incidence of complications in the open group was noted to be higher than in previous reports, and there was no difference noted in overall complication rates between the 2 approaches.[45] Most significantly, recent oncologic assessments comparing open and minimally invasive operations have documented similar lymph node yields,[45–47] inferring that the introduction of minimally invasive procedures has not compromised oncologic outcomes. Reports on quality of life between minimally invasive and open operations have reported mixed results, with some reporting decreased impact on quality of life for the minimally invasive approach,[48] although previous reviews have suggested that long-term quality of life is not necessarily affected by the invasiveness or aggressiveness of the surgical approach.[16,49] Minimally invasive approaches to esophageal resection are clearly a viable alternative with some potential advantages, especially with respect to respiratory complications. Questions regarding the increased potential for conduit necrosis with the minimally invasive approach need to be further assessed.

A recent review of short-term outcomes after esophageal resection in NSQIP hospitals reaffirmed no significant difference in the incidence of complications between the transhiatal and the Ivor Lewis operation. The conclusions highlighted, however, that even with case mix adjustment, hospital performance varied widely and that technical complications should be considered only one component of a much broader assessment of the factors influencing outcomes and the incidence of complications.[24]

MAJOR COMPLICATIONS ASSOCIATED WITH ESOPHAGEAL RESECTION
Respiratory Complications

Respiratory complications have typically been identified as one of the most common components of postoperative esophagectomy morbidity. This is reflected in the recent randomized clinical trial comparing open and minimally invasive esophagectomy, in which the instances of "pulmonary infection" were used as a primary outcome measure.[45] There is no currently standardized format for documenting or stratifying severity of respiratory complications. The section on severity stratification outlines how diverse the presentation of "pneumonia" can be. Pulmonary complications are thought to be responsible for 50% to 65% of mortalities associated with esophagectomy[50,51] and patients who develop pneumonia have a sixfold incidence of perioperative mortality.[14] The incidence of pneumonia has been directly linked to technical complications associated with the surgical procedure.[52] The instance of pneumonia is reported to be lower in open transhiatal operations[36] and, more recently, in minimally invasive procedures.[45]

The high incidence of respiratory complications following esophagectomy is an expression of the major impact the operation has on chest wall, diaphragm, and abdominal wall musculature. The risk of perioperative aspiration and pneumonia is increased in the presence of recurrent nerve injury or dysfunction or in situations of documented poor conduit emptying. Previous studies have failed, however, to document a link between increased aspiration risk and whether or not a pyloric drainage procedure has been done.[53] The risk of aspiration can be decreased by the use of an objective swallowing assessment before the initiation of oral feeding. Berry and colleagues[54] saw the incidence of pneumonia decrease from 18% to 11% associated with this objective assessment.

The effect of neoadjuvant therapy, particularly chemoradiation, on the instance of respiratory complications has been examined, and to date there is no evidence that neoadjuvant therapy increases the incidence of short-term pulmonary or overall morbidity.[43,50,55] Perioperative factors that have been highlighted to decrease the incidence of respiratory morbidity include regional anesthetic techniques, specifically thoracic epidurals,[43,55,56] minimizing perioperative blood loss[57] and perioperative fluid administration,[58] as well as avoidance or early recognition of vocal cord dysfunction.[54,55] Although there is evidence to suggest that major complications impact survival after surgical treatment of esophageal cancer,[11] there is no current evidence that respiratory complications in isolation affect disease-free survivorship.[21]

Chyle Leak

Postoperative leakage of chyle or lymphatic fluid is a well-recognized and challenging clinical complication following esophagectomy. The diagnosis is reasonably straightforward, typically presenting as an increase in output from chest tubes on days 3 through 8, and most commonly associated with the reintroduction of enteric feeding. Clinically significant chyle leaks produce 2 to 4 L per day, and the color of the fluid will change from clear to milky with enteric feeds. If pleural fluid analysis is required, a triglyceride level higher than 100 mg/dL or the presence of chylomicrons within the pleural fluid is considered diagnostic.[59] High-volume chylous leaks are clinically significant because of potential loss of fluids, lymphocytes, and protein that can lead to immunosuppression and malnutrition, increasing the risk of pulmonary and other septic complications.

Significant chylous leaks can be associated with transection of the main duct or leakage from lymphatic collaterals. Previous studies have indicated that the risk of chyle leak is higher following transthoracic compared with transhiatal operations.[60] Mortality associated with a chylous leak has been quoted as high as 50%,[59] although a more recent review from the Netherlands advocating an orchestrated plan of management indicates that mortality can be limited by a systematic approach to treatment at the time of recognition.[61]

When a significant chyle leak is identified, initial response should include discontinuation of enteric feeding and the initiation of total parenteral nutrition (TPN). This typically leads to a significant decrease in output, especially when the situation is associated with chyle leakage from tributaries rather than an interruption of the main duct. If output decreases to less than 500 mL per day, this management approach can be continued and ultimately the patient can be restarted on enteric feeds. If output continues to be high after the initiation of TPN, there are a variety of opinions as to when surgical management should be considered. Some recommend considering surgical intervention if output is more than 2 L per day for 2 consecutive days,[61] whereas others recommend consideration of surgical management if output is more than a liter for 5 consecutive days.[60]

Surgical management can be contemplated using either thoracoscopic or open techniques. Before the operation, a liquid with a high fat content, such as cream, is placed down the nasogastric or jejunostomy tube at least 1 hour before surgical exploration. This helps with the location of the leak at the time of surgery due to the visualization of the characteristic whitish fluid discharge. Various approaches to sealing the leaks have involved the application of hemostatic clips, fibrin glues, or other types of pulmonary sealants. If no specific area of leak can be identified, most surgeons would advocate a "mass ligation" of the main thoracic duct just above the diaphragm by tying off the entire contents of the prevertebral space between the azygos vein and the aorta.

Lymphangiography has historically been considered an alternative management approach, although previous techniques of lymphatic cannulation in the foot and leg are complex procedures not typically done by radiologists in the modern era. Alternative methods of thoracic duct cannulation have been used to manage thoracic duct leaks associated with thoracic trauma and head and neck surgery.[62,63] More recently, a new technical approach was introduced of accessing the lymphatic system through inguinal nodes located under ultrasound and injecting lipiodol (Guerbet LLC, Bloomington, IN), which opacifies the main thoracic duct. The abdominal lymphatic can then be accessed through standard interventional techniques with catheters that can be maneuvered up into the main thoracic duct to localize and embolize the specific tributaries or the main duct with various intravascular glues (**Fig. 1**).[64]

ANASTOMOTIC AND CONDUIT COMPLICATIONS

The opportunity to assess the true incidence and impact of anastomotic leak on outcomes and costs associated with esophagectomy is limited due to the absence of a standardized format for defining a leak and stratifying its severity. There is currently no general agreement as to whether scheduled objective testing most commonly carried out as a scheduled upper gastrointestinal contrast study is indicated and many surgeons will reserve objective assessment of leaks for patients demonstrating concerning clinical signs or changes in output of in-dwelling drains.

If a leak is suspected, the current recommended approach to assessment is a water-soluble contrast study, which we believe is best witnessed by a member of the surgical team. If there is no abnormality, repeated swallows with thin barium and, if clinical suspicion remains, this assessment should be followed immediately by a neck and chest computed tomography (CT) scan. Endoscopic assessment of leaks was previously considered a high-risk procedure in the diagnosis and treatment of leaks and conduit necrosis. Page and colleagues[65] published a report in which they carried out "routine endoscopic assessment" on 79 patients following esophagectomy. There were no procedurally related problems noted, but leaks were diagnosed in 7 patients (9%) and localized "gastric ischemia" was identified in 15 patients, but only 1 of these progressed on to a clinically significant leak.

There is significant variation in the reported leak rate (3.5%–21.0%) following esophagectomy and variation in the reported effect that anastomotic leak has on mortality (0%–35%).[66] There is the impression that, because of refinements in anastomotic technique and overall improvements in perioperative management, that the incidence of

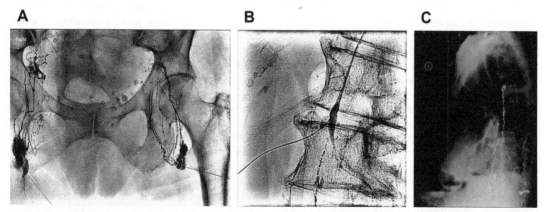

Fig. 1. (*A*) A 77-year-old woman with a 3-L per day chyle leak, 5 days after a transthoracic resection for a YpT1bN0 distal esophageal squamous cell carcinoma. Management with TPN had failed. This radiograph demonstrates the opacification of the patient's inguinal lymph nodes bilaterally with contrast perfusing into abdominal lymphatics. (*B*) Subsequent canalization of the main abdominal thoracic duct under CT guidance. (*C*) Lateral chest radiograph showing the opacification and obstruction of the entire thoracic duct, which led to immediate resolution of the chylous leak.

anastomotic leak following esophagectomy is decreasing.[67]

The manifestation of leaks and the therapeutic response required to treat them are extremely diverse. Leaks can be identified as defects or cavities associated with the anastomosis that are self-limited and drain back into the conduit. They can be defects that connect directly with in-dwelling drains without any indication for systemic sepsis. They can be associated with loculated mediastinal or intrapleural abscesses or can present as leaks draining freely into the pleural cavity. Therapeutic responses to each one of these scenarios can vary from continuing careful clinical monitoring to reoperations requiring drainage, decortication, and either primary repair of the leak or buttressing with a variety of tissues including pericardium, omentum, or muscle flaps. This diversity in presentation and clinical response highlights the need for a uniform reporting system. A recent systematic review by Blencowe and colleagues[10] reviewed more than 57,000 esophageal resections and identified that anastomotic leak was the most commonly reported complication present in 80% of reports but it was associated with a definition in only 28%, and in that group there were 22 different methodologies for defining anastomotic leak.

There are indications that the risk of anastomotic leak is decreased in high-volume centers.[68] Other assessments have indicated that the risk of anastomotic leak is increased with cervical anastomoses.[69] Historically, leaks associated with anastomosis placed in the chest were felt to be more clinically significant, although more up-to-date approaches to treatment appear to have decreased the clinical impact, specifically mortality, of a chest leak.[70] Leak rates do not seem to be specifically affected by the application of either a handsewn or stapled anastomosis[68,71] or by approaches using either transhiatal or transthoracic resections.[72] However, the incidence of anastomotic stricturing is more prevalent in transhiatal operations[73] and in handsewn anastomoses.[71]

The clinical importance of anastomotic leaks and the more severe complication of generalized conduit necrosis is reflected in a series of publications examining the potential role of gastric preconditioning in an attempt to minimize the incidence and impact of these perioperative complications.[74] To date, there has been no significant indication that these preresectional interventions significantly affect the outcomes associated with esophageal resection. The incidence of clinically significant conduit ischemia is variously reported in the range of 1% to 2%.[75,76] Some reports have indicated that the incidence is higher in minimally invasive esophageal resections. The publication by Page and colleagues,[65] using routine endoscopic assessment, demonstrated that regional ischemia in the conduit is a common issue and does not always result in clinically significant leaks. In addition, with the increasing uses of endoscopy for the diagnosis and treatment of esophageal leaks, it is becoming increasingly apparent that many leaks thought to be associated with the anastomosis are actually associated with necrosis of the tip of the gastric conduit.

Endoscopy has also provided a venue for diversifying treatment approaches to, not only localized anastomotic leaks, but also refractory anastomotic strictures (**Fig. 2**).

Expandable metallic or plastic stents can also be successfully used in selected cases of acute anastomotic leak or tip necrosis. **Fig. 3** demonstrates the application of a stent along with interventional treatment to treat an acute anastomotic leak. Endoscopic management of selected leaks can simplify, and potentially shorten, hospital stay, and also reduce costs.

Although the management of esophageal leaks and conduit necrosis remains complex, outcomes will be improved when an experienced surgical team able to apply all operative and endoscopic options for therapy confronts these issues. We have developed a treatment algorithm that can help guide decision making (**Fig. 4**).

OTHER COMPLICATIONS ASSOCIATED WITH ESOPHAGEAL RESECTION
Atrial Fibrillation

Atrial fibrillation is one of the most common complications associated with esophageal resection. In our series of 285 patients, it occurred in 16.8% of patients in the perioperative period.[13] Atrial fibrillation appears to occur more commonly in elderly patients and in patients undergoing neoadjuvant therapy.[77,78] Previous assessments by Murthy and colleagues[79] and Stawicki and colleagues[80] have demonstrated a link between atrial fibrillation and other perioperative complications; specifically, anastomotic leak and pulmonary complications, as well as increased perioperative mortality. Although atrial fibrillation occurs fairly commonly after esophageal resection, its occurrence should stimulate a careful clinical assessment for other complications. Careful reassessment, balancing of electrolytes, and treatment with antiarrhythmics and even defibrillation are indicated, as the effect of atrial fibrillation on conduit profusion is currently incompletely understood. At the present time, there are early indications that prophylactic amiodarone[81] and laparoscopic surgery[82] may decrease the incidence of atrial fibrillation associated with esophagectomy.

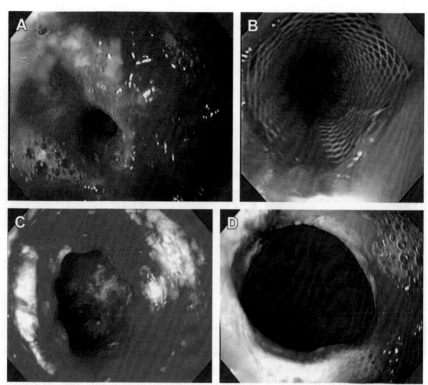

Fig. 2. Treatment of chronic refractory anastomotic stricture with temporary stent. Figure highlights a 65-year-old woman who developed dysphagia 4 months following transthoracic esophagectomy with cervical anastomosis. (*A*) Endoscopy of a tight anastomotic stricture that had been treated with dilation 4 times, the last 2 including injection of Kenalog (Bristol-Myers Squibb Company, Princeton, NJ). (*B*) Endoscopy following the insertion of a Polyflex stent (Boston Scientific, Natick, MA). (*C*) Endoscopic picture immediately following stent removal 4 weeks after insertion. (*D*) Anastomosis 1 year following treatment with the remodeling of the perianastomotic scar resulting in a widely patent anastomosis.

Recurrent Laryngeal Nerve Injury

The incidence of recurrent nerve injury is variously reported to be between 2% and 20%.[83] These injuries are more often associated with cervical anastomoses and 3-field lymph node dissections. The occurrence of a recurrent laryngeal nerve palsy or injury increases the incidence of perioperative pulmonary complications.[54,55] Injury to the recurrent nerve can occur in relation to the removal of bulky proximal tumors, extensive lymph node dissections, and retraction injuries, especially in the neck. Vocal cord dysfunction following esophagectomy can demonstrate spontaneous resolution in up to 40% of cases.[84] However, suspicion of vocal cord dysfunction should initiate an objective swallowing evaluation[54] and can ultimately be dealt with by either temporary or permanent vocal cord medialization.[83]

Postesophagectomy Delirium

Historically, many surgeons have looked on delirium as a manifestation of other complications,

particularly sepsis. However, we have recently demonstrated that when critically assessed, delirium occurs in up to 9.2% of patients after esophagectomy and either presents in isolation or precedes other complications in 67% of cases. The incidence of delirium is higher in older patients and with the use of sedative medication in the ICU setting.[85] The occurrence of delirium leads to increased incidence of pulmonary complications, length of hospital stay, and overall hospital costs.[86] A proactive approach to identifying patients at risk and identifying the early signs of delirium can facilitate intervention, specifically with increased mobility protocols, family contact, and potentially the use of bright light therapy.[87]

METHODS OF AFFECTING THE INCIDENCE OF COMPLICATIONS ASSOCIATED WITH ESOPHAGECTOMY

Any current audit of quality outcome measures associated with esophagectomy will inevitably have complications as a major focus. Malnutrition

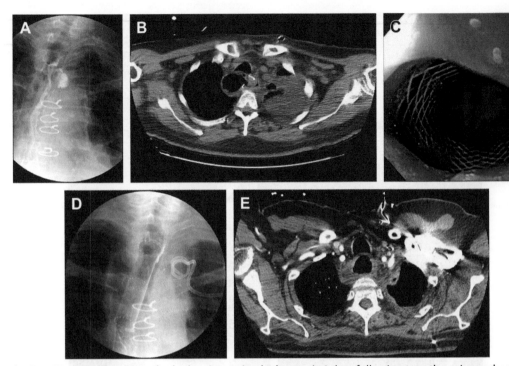

Fig. 3. A 71-year-old patient who had an increasing leukocytosis 4 days following transthoracic esophagectomy with cervical anastomosis. (*A*) A gastrografin swallow confirming an anastomotic leak. (*B*) Subsequent CT scan demonstrating the leak communicating with a fluid collection in the apex of the right chest. (*C*) Endoscopy confirming no significant evidence of conduit necrosis, and a Polyflex stent was inserted. (*D*) Radiograph demonstrating the interventional radiology–placed drain in the apical fluid collection that was placed the same day as stent insertion. (*E*) CT scan of patient 1 month following treatment. Drain was removed 5 days following insertion, and the stent was removed after 3 weeks. The patient was discharged on postoperative day 10 and was able to maintain oral intake throughout the postoperative period.

is a common sequela associated with the presentation and treatment of esophageal cancer and it is currently estimated that up to 80% of patients manifest a degree of malnutrition at the time of diagnosis. Malnutrition is associated with increased incidence of complications, including sepsis, pulmonary complications, and mortality. A working definition[88] of malnutrition currently includes the following:

- Body mass index (BMI) lower than 18.5 kg/m^2
- Unintentional weight loss of more than 10% within the past 3 to 6 months
- BMI lower than 20 kg/m^2 and unintentional weight loss of more than 5% within the past 3 to 6 months

The percentage of obese patients undergoing esophageal resection is increasing, and these patients can also present malnourished. Although obesity does not appear to be a risk factor for complications, obese patients who are diabetic are at increased risk for atrial fibrillation and anastomotic leaks.[89] If malnutrition is suspected at the time of diagnosis, it is currently recommended that the patient receive 10 to 14 days of enteric nutrition preoperatively[90] with jejunal feeding tubes being preferred over nasojejunal or percutaneous endoscopic gastrostomy tubes.

In the perioperative setting, there are increasing indications that various approaches to immunonutrition, specifically those containing polyunsaturated Omega 3 fatty acids, arginine, glutamine, nucleotides, and antioxidant micronutrients, including vitamins E and C, beta-carotene, zinc, and selenium, may improve recovery and limit complications. There are randomized controlled trials that have demonstrated a reduction in infectious complications when immunonutrition is used for 5 to 7 days preoperatively. It may also lead to an overall decrease in length of stay.[91–93]

Neoadjuvant therapy, specifically chemoradiation, is becoming a routine component of therapy for patients with locoregional esophageal cancer. In addition to the standard obstructive issues that patients with esophageal cancer must confront, radiation combined with chemotherapy can produce additional problems of mucositis, esophagitis, nausea, and decreased appetite, all of which can

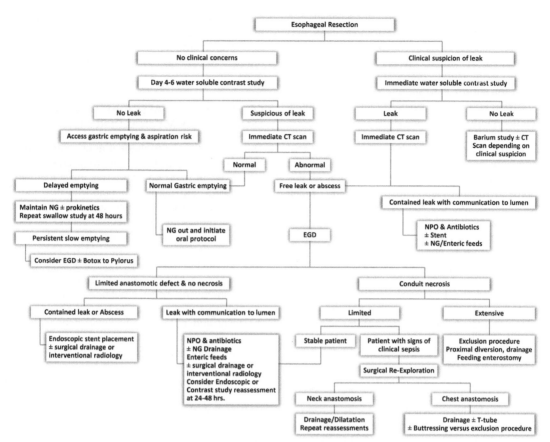

Fig. 4. Algorithm for diagnosis and management of postesophagectomy anastomic leaks. EGD, esophagogastro-duodenoscopy; NG, nasogastric; NPO, nothing by mouth. (*From* Low DE. Diagnosis and management of anastomotic leaks after esophagectomy. J Gastrointest Surg 2011;15(8):1320; with permission.)

compound the potential for malnutrition. Dietary consultation throughout radiotherapy has been shown to improve recovery and quality of life in patients undergoing trimodality therapy.[94] There are some preliminary publications indicating that temporary plastic or metallic removable stents can be used to palliate dysphagia during neoadjuvant chemoradiotherapy.[95] Issues with this approach center around problems with stent migration, and the question as to whether these stents should be removed on a scheduled basis or left in place until surgical resection. A retrospective review comparing plastic removable stents and feeding jejunostomies demonstrated that both could provide improvement in nutritional status with significant improvement in dysphagia in the stent group and no significant difference in complication rates associated with insertion.[96] There is no current consensus regarding the routine application of jejunostomy tubes following esophagectomy, although many surgeons use them to ensure postoperative nutrition and help facilitate adherence to fast-tracking or standardized recovery protocols.

There is also evidence to suggest that early postoperative enteral feedings can decrease the incidence of life-threatening complications.[97]

Perioperative issues assessed for their potential to improve recovery and decrease complications include a more conservative approach to perioperative fluid management. These approaches have been documented to improve outcomes in major intra-abdominal operations,[98] and 2 specific publications associated with esophagectomy demonstrated that a more restrictive approach to perioperative fluids can improve early extubation rates and decrease overall and, specifically, pulmonary complications.[58,99]

Perioperative pain control remains a critical issue, especially with an operation as potentially extensive as esophageal resection. A meta-analysis of abdominal and thoracic operations demonstrated that thoracic epidurals could contribute to early extubation, decrease pulmonary complications, and promote an earlier return of bowel function, which facilitates expeditious resumption of enteric feeding.[100] There are also suggestions that thoracic epidural analgesia can reduce the incidence of anastomotic leak and improve microcirculation to the conduit.[101,102] Other effective postoperative pain approaches include extrapleural intercostal catheters that have been shown, in a randomized controlled trial, to provide equivalent results to thoracic epidurals with respect to postthoracotomy pain and recovery of pulmonary function.[103] We currently recommend that when thoracic epidurals are used, that immediate postoperative pain issues should not be accompanied by bolusing the epidural, as this approach routinely leads to hypotension, which can affect gastric conduit perfusion. We recommend modifying the standard rate of the epidural infusion and selectively using vasopressors to maintain a mean arterial pressure higher than 70 mm Hg in the immediate postoperative period.

For too long, surgeons have focused on the operation as the key issue under their control regarding improving outcomes, including morbidity associated with esophagectomy. Although meticulous surgery remains central to quality outcomes in major cancer surgery, standardized clinical pathways and enhanced recovery programs are now recognized as a potential framework for impacting the entire treatment and recovery process. Standardized clinical pathways applied in thoracic surgery have demonstrated significant reductions in mortality rates, length of stay, and costs.[104] Enhanced recovery programs specifically developed for esophagectomy have demonstrated similar improvements in mortality, length of stay, and complications.[105] Fast-tracking programs have been developed for esophagectomy, but tend to focus on only the immediate operative and recovery time frames.[106] We developed a standardized clinical pathway in 1991 that covers all aspects of the patient's journey from the time of the referral until 3 years following resection. It has undergone 5 revisions to date, and the construction and revision of the pathway involves all the caregivers who work with a patient throughout staging, medical and surgical therapy, and recovery. Thoracic oncology nurse coordinators are the most important individual component of the pathway, as they serve as the focal point for coordination of the patient's journey and maintaining communication with caregivers, patients, and family members. This approach has facilitated significant decreases in length of stay, perioperative blood loss, and major complications, including anastomotic leak. It has also provided an infrastructure, which in 340 consecutive patients resulted in a perioperative mortality rate of less than 1%.[107] We also recently demonstrated that the concepts contained in these structured pathways can be transplanted into different hospitals and medical systems with significant short-term improvements in extubation rates, first-day mobilization, length of stay, and complication rates.[108]

COMPLICATIONS ASSOCIATED WITH ESOPHAGECTOMY IN ELDERLY PATIENTS

The incidence of esophageal adenocarcinoma is increasing worldwide but more prominently in elderly white male patients. This inevitably leads to medical and surgical oncologists needing to provide a balanced treatment approach in patients with nonmetastatic esophageal cancer in more advanced age groups. Viklund and colleagues[68] demonstrated that older age can be associated with increased risk of complications. A recent systematic review confirms that elderly patients are at increased risk for pulmonary and cardiac complications, as well as increased perioperative mortality and potentially reduced cancer-related 5-year survivorship.[109] An assessment in 2009 using the Surveillance, Epidemiology, and End Results (SEER) Medicare database comparing esophagectomy and definitive chemoradiation for early-stage esophageal cancer in older patients demonstrated that in carefully selected populations, esophagectomy can be associated with improved survivorship compared with definitive chemoradiation.[110] There are now 3 single-institution series assessing the results of esophagectomy in patients older than 80. Moskovitz and colleagues[111] demonstrated that a cohort of 31 patients older than 80 had higher mortality (19.4% vs 5.8%) and longer length of stay (26 days vs 16.4 days) in addition to worse long-term survival compared with younger patients. However, 2 other more recent articles by Morita and colleagues[112] and Markar and Low[113] demonstrated that carefully selected octogenarian patients demonstrated a higher incidence of overall complications, but no mortalities occurred in the over-80 populations in either of these studies, and there was no overall difference in survivorship. These data would suggest that patients should not be denied access to therapy simply on the basis of their age, but should be reviewed by an experienced high-volume center and have a careful assessment of their overall physiologic status before treatment decision making.

REFERENCES

1. Finks JF, Osborne NH, Birkmeyer JD. Trends in hospital volume and operative mortality for high-risk surgery. N Engl J Med 2011;364:2128–37.

2. Markar SR, Karthikesalingam A, Thrumurthy S, et al. Volume-outcome relationship in surgery for esophageal malignancy: systematic review and meta-analysis 2000-2011. J Gastrointest Surg 2012;16:1055–63.

3. Wright CD, Kucharczuk JC, O'Brien SM, et al. Predictors of major morbidity and mortality after esophagectomy for esophageal cancer: a Society of Thoracic Surgeons General Thoracic Surgery Database risk adjustment model. J Thorac Cardiovasc Surg 2009;137:587–95.

4. Enestvedt CK, Perry KA, Kim C, et al. Trends in the management of esophageal carcinoma based on provider volume: treatment practices of 618 esophageal surgeons. Dis Esophagus 2010;23:136–44.

5. The Leapfrog Group Evidence-based Hospital Referral Fact Sheet. 2008. Available at: http://www.leapfroggroup.org/media/file/Leapfrog-Evidence-Based_Hospital_Referral_Fact_Sheet.pdf. Accessed January 18, 2013.

6. Kohn GP, Galanko JA, Meyers MO, et al. National trends in esophageal surgery—are outcomes as good as we believe? J Gastrointest Surg 2009;13:1900–10.

7. van Lanschot JJ, Hulscher JB, Buskens CJ, et al. Hospital volume and hospital mortality for esophagectomy. Cancer 2001;91:1574–8.

8. Dunst CM, Swanstrom LL. Minimally invasive esophagectomy. J Gastrointest Surg 2010;14(Suppl 1):S108–14.

9. Bailey SH, Bull DA, Harpole DH, et al. Outcomes after esophagectomy: a ten-year prospective cohort. Ann Thorac Surg 2003;75:217–22.

10. Blencowe NS, Strong S, McNair AG, et al. Reporting of short-term clinical outcomes after esophagectomy: a systematic review. Ann Surg 2012;255:658–66.

11. Rizk NP, Bach PB, Schrag D, et al. The impact of complications on outcomes after resection for esophageal and gastroesophageal junction carcinoma. J Am Coll Surg 2004;198:42–50.

12. Schieman C, Wigle DA, Deschamps C, et al. Patterns of operative mortality following esophagectomy. Dis Esophagus 2012;25:645–51.

13. Carrott PW, Markar SR, Kuppusamy MK, et al. Accordion severity grading system: assessment of relationship between costs, length of hospital stay, and survival in patients with complications after esophagectomy for cancer. J Am Coll Surg 2012;215:331–6.

14. Hii MW, Smithers BM, Gotley DC, et al. Impact of postoperative morbidity on long-term survival after oesophagectomy. Br J Surg 2013;100:95–104.

15. Viklund P, Lindblad M, Lagergren J. Influence of surgery-related factors on quality of life after esophageal or cardia cancer resection. World J Surg 2005;29:841–8.

16. Scarpa M, Valente S, Alfieri R, et al. Systematic review of health-related quality of life after esophagectomy for esophageal cancer. World J Gastroenterol 2011;17:4660–74.

17. Derogar M, Orsini N, Sadr-Azodi O, et al. Influence of major postoperative complications on health-related quality of life among long-term survivors of esophageal cancer surgery. J Clin Oncol 2012;30:1615–9.

18. Kalish RL, Daley J, Duncan CC, et al. Costs of potential complications of care for major surgery patients. Am J Med Qual 1995;10:48–54.

19. Lerut T, Moons J, Coosemans W, et al. Postoperative complications after transthoracic esophagectomy for cancer of the esophagus and gastroesophageal junction are correlated with early cancer recurrence: role of systematic grading of complications using the modified Clavien classification. Ann Surg 2009;250:798–807.

20. Rutegard M, Lagergren P, Rouvelas I, et al. Surgical complications and long-term survival after esophagectomy for cancer in a nationwide Swedish cohort study. Eur J Surg Oncol 2012;38:555–61.

21. D'Annoville T, D'Journo XB, Trousse D, et al. Respiratory complications after oesophagectomy for cancer do not affect disease-free survival. Eur J Cardiothorac Surg 2012;41:e66–73.

22. Bruce J, Russell EM, Mollison J, et al. The measurement and monitoring of surgical adverse events. Health Technol Assess 2001;5:1–194.

23. Hanna GB, Arya S, Markar SR. Variation in the standard of minimally invasive esophagectomy for cancer—systematic review. Semin Thorac Cardiovasc Surg 2012;24:176–87.

24. Merkow RP, Bilimoria KY, McCarter MD, et al. Short-term outcomes after esophagectomy at 164 American College of Surgeons National Surgical Quality Improvement Program Hospitals: effect of operative approach and hospital-level variation. Arch Surg 2012;147:1009–16.

25. Veen EJ, Steenbruggen J, Roukema JA. Classifying surgical complications: a critical appraisal. Arch Surg 2005;140:1078–83.

26. Fleming ST. Complications, adverse events, and iatrogenesis: classifications and quality of care measurement issues. Clin Perform Qual Health Care 1996;4:137–47.

27. Dindo D, Demartines N, Clavien PA. Classification of surgical complications: a new proposal with evaluation in a cohort of 6336 patients and results of a survey. Ann Surg 2004;240:205–13.

28. Strasberg SM, Linehan DC, Hawkins WG. The Accordion severity grading system of surgical complications. Ann Surg 2009;250:177–86.

29. Low DE, Kuppusamy M, Hashimoto Y, et al. Comparing complications of esophagectomy and pancreaticoduodenectomy and potential impact

on hospital systems utilizing the Accordion severity grading system. J Gastrointest Surg 2010;14: 1646–52.

30. van der Sluis PC, Ruurda JP, van der Horst S, et al. Robot-assisted minimally invasive thoraco-laparoscopic esophagectomy versus open transthoracic esophagectomy for resectable esophageal cancer, a randomized controlled trial (ROBOT trial). Trials 2012;13:230.

31. Copeland GP, Jones D, Walters M. POSSUM: a scoring system for surgical audit. Br J Surg 1991; 78:355–60.

32. Reynolds PQ, Sanders NW, Schildcrout JS, et al. Expansion of the surgical Apgar score across all surgical subspecialties as a means to predict post-operative mortality. Anesthesiology 2011;114: 1305–12.

33. Haga Y, Wada Y, Takeuchi H, et al. Prediction of anastomotic leak and its prognosis in digestive surgery. World J Surg 2011;35:716–22.

34. Trotti A, Colevas AD, Setser A, et al. CTCAE v3.0: development of a comprehensive grading system for the adverse effects of cancer treatment. Semin Radiat Oncol 2003;13:176–81.

35. Grotenhuis BA, van Hagen P, Reitsma JB, et al. Validation of a nomogram predicting complications after esophagectomy for cancer. Ann Thorac Surg 2010;90:920–5.

36. Hulscher JB, van Sandick JW, de Boer AG, et al. Extended transthoracic resection compared with limited transhiatal resection for adenocarcinoma of the esophagus. N Engl J Med 2002;347:1662–9.

37. Omloo JM, Lagarde SM, Hulscher JB, et al. Extended transthoracic resection compared with limited transhiatal resection for adenocarcinoma of the mid/distal esophagus: five-year survival of a randomized clinical trial. Ann Surg 2007;246: 992–1000.

38. Hulscher JB, van Lanschot JJ. Individualised surgical treatment of patients with an adenocarcinoma of the distal oesophagus or gastro-oesophageal junction. Dig Surg 2005;22:130–4.

39. Connors RC, Reuben BC, Neumayer LA, et al. Comparing outcomes after transthoracic and transhiatal esophagectomy: a 5-year prospective cohort of 17,395 patients. J Am Coll Surg 2007; 205:735–40.

40. Rentz J, Bull D, Harpole D, et al. Transthoracic versus transhiatal esophagectomy: a prospective study of 945 patients. J Thorac Cardiovasc Surg 2003;125:1114–20.

41. Boone J, Livestro DP, Elias SG, et al. International survey on esophageal cancer: part I surgical techniques. Dis Esophagus 2009;22:195–202.

42. National Oesophago-Gastric Cancer Audit. An audit of the care received by people with Oesophago-Gastric Cancer in England and Wales.

Third Annual Report 2010. The Information Centre, NHS. Available at: https://catalogue.ic.nhs.uk/publications/clinical/oesophago-gastric/nati-clin-audi-supp-prog-oeso-gast-canc-2010/clin-audi-supp-prog-oeso-gast-2010-rep1.pdf. Accessed February 1, 2013.

43. Zingg U, Smithers BM, Gotley DC, et al. Factors associated with postoperative pulmonary morbidity after esophagectomy for cancer. Ann Surg Oncol 2011;18:1460–8.

44. Briez N, Piessen G, Torres F, et al. Effects of hybrid minimally invasive oesophagectomy on major post-operative pulmonary complications. Br J Surg 2012;99:1547–53.

45. Biere SS, van Berge Henegouwen MI, Maas KW, et al. Minimally invasive versus open oesophagectomy for patients with oesophageal cancer: a multicentre, open-label, randomised controlled trial. Lancet 2012;379:1887–92.

46. Palanivelu C, Prakash A, Senthilkumar R, et al. Minimally invasive esophagectomy: thoracoscopic mobilization of the esophagus and mediastinal lymphadenectomy in prone position—experience of 130 patients. J Am Coll Surg 2006;203:7–16.

47. Singhal R, Pallan L, Taniere P, et al. Oncological acceptability of laparoscopic surgery for locally advanced oesophageal adenocarcinoma. Br J Surg 2008;95(Suppl 3):1–84.

48. Parameswaran R, Blazeby JM, Hughes R, et al. Health-related quality of life after minimally invasive oesophagectomy. Br J Surg 2010;97:525–31.

49. Rutegard M, Lagergren J, Rouvelas I, et al. Population-based study of surgical factors in relation to health-related quality of life after oesophageal cancer resection. Br J Surg 2008;95:592–601.

50. Atkins BZ, Shah AS, Hutcheson KA, et al. Reducing hospital morbidity and mortality following esophagectomy. Ann Thorac Surg 2004;78:1170–6.

51. Bakhos CT, Fabian T, Oyasiji TO, et al. Impact of the surgical technique on pulmonary morbidity after esophagectomy. Ann Thorac Surg 2012;93:221–6.

52. Ferri LE, Law S, Wong KH, et al. The influence of technical complications on postoperative outcome and survival after esophagectomy. Ann Surg Oncol 2006;13:557–64.

53. Urschel JD, Blewett CJ, Young JE, et al. Pyloric drainage (pyloroplasty) or no drainage in gastric reconstruction after esophagectomy: a meta-analysis of randomized controlled trials. Dig Surg 2002;19:160–4.

54. Berry MF, Atkins BZ, Tong BC, et al. A comprehensive evaluation for aspiration after esophagectomy reduces the incidence of postoperative pneumonia. J Thorac Cardiovasc Surg 2010;140: 1266–71.

55. Dumont P, Wihlm JM, Hentz JG, et al. Respiratory complications after surgical treatment

of esophageal cancer. A study of 309 patients according to the type of resection. Eur J Cardiothorac Surg 1995;9:539–43.

56. Tsui SL, Law S, Fok M, et al. Postoperative analgesia reduces mortality and morbidity after esophagectomy. Am J Surg 1997;173:472–8.

57. Law S, Wong KH, Kwok KF, et al. Predictive factors for postoperative pulmonary complications and mortality after esophagectomy for cancer. Ann Surg 2004;240:791–800.

58. Kita T, Mammoto T, Kishi Y. Fluid management and postoperative respiratory disturbances in patients with transthoracic esophagectomy for carcinoma. J Clin Anesth 2002;14:252–6.

59. Merrigan BA, Winter DC, O'Sullivan GC. Chylothorax. Br J Surg 1997;84:15–20.

60. Cerfolio RJ, Allen MS, Deschamps C, et al. Postoperative chylothorax. J Thorac Cardiovasc Surg 1996;112:1361–5.

61. Lagarde SM, Omloo JM, de Jong K, et al. Incidence and management of chyle leakage after esophagectomy. Ann Thorac Surg 2005;80:449–54.

62. van Goor AT, Kroger R, Klomp HM, et al. Introduction of lymphangiography and percutaneous embolization of the thoracic duct in a stepwise approach to the management of chylous fistulas. Head Neck 2007;29:1017–23.

63. Itkin M, Kucharczuk JC, Kwak A, et al. Nonoperative thoracic duct embolization for traumatic thoracic duct leak: experience in 109 patients. J Thorac Cardiovasc Surg 2010;139:584–9.

64. Nadolski GJ, Itkin M. Feasibility of ultrasound-guided intranodal lymphangiogram for thoracic duct embolization. J Vasc Interv Radiol 2012;23: 613–6.

65. Page RD, Asmat A, McShane J, et al. Routine endoscopy to detect anastomotic leakage after esophagectomy. Ann Thorac Surg 2013;95:292–8.

66. Sarela AI, Tolan DJ, Harris K, et al. Anastomotic leakage after esophagectomy for cancer: a mortality-free experience. J Am Coll Surg 2008; 206:516–23.

67. Lerut T, Coosemans W, Decker G, et al. Anastomotic complications after esophagectomy. Dig Surg 2002;19:92–8.

68. Viklund P, Lindblad M, Lu M, et al. Risk factors for complications after esophageal cancer resection: a prospective population-based study in Sweden. Ann Surg 2006;243:204–11.

69. Biere SS, Maas KW, Cuesta MA, et al. Cervical or thoracic anastomosis after esophagectomy for cancer: a systematic review and meta-analysis. Dig Surg 2011;28:29–35.

70. Martin LW, Swisher SG, Hofstetter W, et al. Intrathoracic leaks following esophagectomy are no longer associated with increased mortality. Ann Surg 2005;242:392–9.

71. Ercan S, Rice TW, Murthy SC, et al. Does esophagogastric anastomotic technique influence the outcome of patients with esophageal cancer? J Thorac Cardiovasc Surg 2005;129:623–31.

72. Chu KM, Law SY, Fok M, et al. A prospective randomized comparison of transhiatal and transthoracic resection for lower-third esophageal carcinoma. Am J Surg 1997;174:320–4.

73. Chang AC, Ji H, Birkmeyer NJ, et al. Outcomes after transhiatal and transthoracic esophagectomy for cancer. Ann Thorac Surg 2008;85:424–9.

74. Holscher AH, Schneider PM, Gutschow C, et al. Laparoscopic ischemic conditioning of the stomach for esophageal replacement. Ann Surg 2007; 245:241–6.

75. Griffin SM, Shaw IH, Dresner SM. Early complications after Ivor Lewis subtotal esophagectomy with two-field lymphadenectomy: risk factors and management. J Am Coll Surg 2002;194:285–97.

76. Orringer MB, Marshall B, Chang AC, et al. Two thousand transhiatal esophagectomies: changing trends, lessons learned. Ann Surg 2007;246: 363–72.

77. Ma JY, Wang Y, Zhao YF, et al. Atrial fibrillation after surgery for esophageal carcinoma: clinical and prognostic significance. World J Gastroenterol 2006;12:449–52.

78. Rao VP, Addae-Boateng E, Barua A, et al. Age and neo-adjuvant chemotherapy increase the risk of atrial fibrillation following oesophagectomy. Eur J Cardiothorac Surg 2012;42:438–43.

79. Murthy SC, Law S, Whooley BP, et al. Atrial fibrillation after esophagectomy is a marker for postoperative morbidity and mortality. J Thorac Cardiovasc Surg 2003;126:1162–7.

80. Stawicki SP, Prosciak MP, Gerlach AT, et al. Atrial fibrillation after esophagectomy: an indicator of postoperative morbidity. Gen Thorac Cardiovasc Surg 2011;59:399–405.

81. Tisdale JE, Wroblewski HA, Wall DS, et al. A randomized, controlled study of amiodarone for prevention of atrial fibrillation after transthoracic esophagectomy. J Thorac Cardiovasc Surg 2010; 140:45–51.

82. Turaga KK, Shah KU, Neill EO, et al. Does laparoscopic surgery decrease the risk of atrial fibrillation after foregut surgery? Surg Endosc 2009;23:204–8.

83. Raymond D. Complications of esophagectomy. Surg Clin North Am 2012;92:1299–313.

84. Baba M, Natsugoe S, Shimada M, et al. Does hoarseness of voice from recurrent nerve paralysis after esophagectomy for carcinoma influence patient quality of life? J Am Coll Surg 1999;188:231–6.

85. Takeuchi M, Takeuchi H, Fujisawa D, et al. Incidence and risk factors of postoperative delirium in patients with esophageal cancer. Ann Surg Oncol 2012;19:3963–70.

86. Markar S, Smith I, Karthikesalingam A, et al. The clinical and economic cost of delirium following surgical resection for esophageal malignancy. Ann Surg 2013;258(1):77–81.

87. Ono H, Taguchi T, Kido Y, et al. The usefulness of bright light therapy for patients after oesophagectomy. Intensive Crit Care Nurs 2011;27:158–66.

88. Allum WH, Blazeby JM, Griffin SM, et al. Guidelines for the management of oesophageal and gastric cancer. Gut 2011;60:1449–72.

89. Kayani B, Okabayashi K, Ashrafian H, et al. Does obesity affect outcomes in patients undergoing esophagectomy for cancer? A meta-analysis. World J Surg 2012;36:1785–95.

90. Weimann A, Braga M, Harsanyi L, et al. ESPEN guidelines on enteral nutrition: surgery including organ transplantation. Clin Nutr 2006;25:224–44.

91. Gianotti L, Braga M, Nespoli L, et al. A randomized controlled trial of preoperative oral supplementation with a specialized diet in patients with gastrointestinal cancer. Gastroenterology 2002;122:1763–70.

92. Braga M, Gianotti L, Vignali A, et al. Preoperative oral arginine and n-3 fatty acid supplementation improves the immunometabolic host response and outcome after colorectal resection for cancer. Surgery 2002;132:805–14.

93. Mariette C, De Botton ML, Piessen G. Surgery in esophageal and gastric cancer patients: what is the role for nutrition support in your daily practice? Ann Surg Oncol 2012;19:2128–34.

94. Isenring EA, Capra S, Bauer JD. Nutrition intervention is beneficial in oncology outpatients receiving radiotherapy to the gastrointestinal or head and neck area. Br J Cancer 2004;91:447–52.

95. Brown RE, Abbas AE, Ellis S, et al. A prospective phase II evaluation of esophageal stenting for neoadjuvant therapy for esophageal cancer: optimal performance and surgical safety. J Am Coll Surg 2011;212:582–8.

96. Siddiqui AA, Glynn C, Loren D, et al. Self-expanding plastic esophageal stents versus jejunostomy tubes for the maintenance of nutrition during neoadjuvant chemoradiation therapy in patients with esophageal cancer: a retrospective study. Dis Esophagus 2009;22:216–22.

97. Fujita T, Daiko H, Nishimura M. Early enteral nutrition reduces the rate of life-threatening complications after thoracic esophagectomy in patients with esophageal cancer. Eur Surg Res 2012;48:79–84.

98. Nisanevich V, Felsenstein I, Almogy G, et al. Effect of intraoperative fluid management on outcome after intraabdominal surgery. Anesthesiology 2005;103:25–32.

99. Neal JM, Wilcox RT, Allen HW, et al. Near-total esophagectomy: the influence of standardized multimodal management and intraoperative fluid restriction. Reg Anesth Pain Med 2003;28:328–34.

100. Popping DM, Elia N, Marret E, et al. Protective effects of epidural analgesia on pulmonary complications after abdominal and thoracic surgery: a meta-analysis. Arch Surg 2008;143:990–9.

101. Lazar G, Kaszaki J, Abraham S, et al. Thoracic epidural anesthesia improves the gastric microcirculation during experimental gastric tube formation. Surgery 2003;134:799–805.

102. Michelet P, D'Journo XB, Roch A, et al. Perioperative risk factors for anastomotic leakage after esophagectomy: influence of thoracic epidural analgesia. Chest 2005;128:3461–6.

103. Kaiser AM, Zollinger A, De Lorenzi D, et al. Prospective, randomized comparison of extrapleural versus epidural analgesia for postthoracotomy pain. Ann Thorac Surg 1998;66:367–72.

104. Zehr KJ, Dawson PB, Yang SC, et al. Standardized clinical care pathways for major thoracic cases reduce hospital costs. Ann Thorac Surg 1998;66:914–9.

105. Munitiz V, Martinez-de-Haro LF, Ortiz A, et al. Effectiveness of a written clinical pathway for enhanced recovery after transthoracic (Ivor Lewis) oesophagectomy. Br J Surg 2010;97:714–8.

106. Cerfolio RJ, Bryant AS, Bass CS, et al. Fast tracking after Ivor Lewis esophagogastrectomy. Chest 2004;126:1187–94.

107. Low DE, Kunz S, Schembre D, et al. Esophagectomy—it's not just about mortality anymore: standardized perioperative clinical pathways improve outcomes in patients with esophageal cancer. J Gastrointest Surg 2007;11:1395–402.

108. Preston SR, Markar SR, Baker CR, et al. Impact of a multidisciplinary standardized clinical pathway on perioperative outcomes in patients with oesophageal cancer. Br J Surg 2013;100:105–12.

109. Markar SR, Karthikesalingam A, Thrumurthy S, et al. Systematic review and pooled analysis assessing the association between elderly age and outcome following surgical resection of esophageal malignancy. Dis Esophagus 2012;26(3):250–62.

110. Abrams JA, Buono DL, Strauss J, et al. Esophagectomy compared with chemoradiation for early stage esophageal cancer in the elderly. Cancer 2009;115:4924–33.

111. Moskovitz AH, Rizk NP, Venkatraman E, et al. Mortality increases for octogenarians undergoing esophagogastrectomy for esophageal cancer. Ann Thorac Surg 2006;82:2031–6.

112. Morita M, Egashira A, Yoshida R, et al. Esophagectomy in patients 80 years of age and older with carcinoma of the thoracic esophagus. J Gastroenterol 2008;43:345–51.

113. Markar SR, Low DE. Physiology, not chronology, dictates outcomes after esophagectomy for esophageal cancer: outcomes in patients 80 years and older. Ann Surg Oncol 2012;16(5):1055–63.

Chemoradiation for Esophageal Cancer

Mariela A. Blum, MD[a], Takashi Taketa, MD[a],
Kazuki Sudo, MD[a], Roopma Wadhwa, MD[a],
Heath D. Skinner, MD, PhD[b], Jaffer A. Ajani, MD[a,*]

KEYWORDS

* Esophageal carcinoma * Definitive chemoradiation * Radiotherapy * Multimodality therapy

KEY POINTS

* There is a subset of esophageal cancer patients who seem to benefit from definitive chemoradiation. Selection of such patients improves with the multidisciplinary interactions with colleagues of all relevant disciplines on a regular basis.
* Identifying patients with high probability of a complete pathologic response (pathCR) through predictive models that can incorporate clinical parameters and biomarkers is challenging and is an area of active research.
* In the future, better understanding of the molecular biology involved in response should lead to rationally designed clinical trials targeting those patients who are at risk for treatment failure.

INTRODUCTION

Globally, esophageal cancer (EC) is the sixth leading cause of cancer death, with an estimated 482,000 new cases and 407,000 deaths in 2008.[1,2] The diagnosis of EC heralds an ominous prognosis, as more than half of the patients have advanced or inoperable disease. Because screening strategies are not well developed, EC is often diagnosed in symptomatic patients; thus, only 30% of patients will have localized disease at diagnosis,[3] and the overall 5-year survival for those able to undergo resection is approximately 47%, with even worse survival rates in those patients unable to undergo primary resection.[4] The 5-year survival rates for localized EC (LEC) have improved recently, owing to the addition of preoperative treatment and better management of morbidities resulting from surgery.

The 2 most common histologic subtypes of EC are squamous cell carcinoma, most prevalent in the Caspian littoral and China,[5,6] and adenocarcinoma, increasing in incidence in the western countries since 1970.[7,8]

The treatment of LEC is challenging. Factors involved in the treatment decision include baseline clinical stage, location of the primary, and, in some instances, histology. Some geographic variations in approach are evident based on the patterns of practice, and likely reflect bias due to the body habitus of the patient population, age, and the dominant histology. Associated comorbid conditions are often incorporated in the decision-making process for the recommendation of a specific therapy. Among many prognostic factors, lymph node involvement carries the highest impact in prognosticating survival.[9] Historically, surgical resection of LEC has been the most

Disclosures: The authors have nothing to disclose.
[a] Department of Gastrointestinal Medical Oncology, The University of Texas MD Anderson Cancer Center, 1515 Holcombe Boulevard, Houston, TX 77030, USA; [b] Department of Radiation Oncology, The University of Texas MD Anderson Cancer Center, 1515 Holcombe Boulevard, Houston, TX 77030, USA
* Corresponding author. The University of Texas MD Anderson Cancer Center, 1515 Holcombe Boulevard, Unit 426, Houston, TX 77030.
E-mail address: jajani@mdanderson.org

Thorac Surg Clin 23 (2013) 551–558
http://dx.doi.org/10.1016/j.thorsurg.2013.07.006
1547-4127/13/$ – see front matter © 2013 Elsevier Inc. All rights reserved.

common primary approach, but in most patients, primary surgery results in dismal outcomes.[10]

Over the last several years, several clinical trials have been completed in EC. Preoperative chemotherapy and preoperative chemoradiation have been the predominant strategies to improve surgical outcome, while bimodality treatment (definitive chemotherapy and radiation) has been reserved for patients with cervical tumors or patients with LEC who are medically inoperable or have technically unresectable disease.

The purpose of this article is to discuss the representative published data forming the basis of contemporary recommendations for LEC.

Definitive Chemoradiotherapy Versus Radiotherapy Alone

Based on the encouraging data using concurrent chemoradiation in patients with anal cancer,[11] several prospective studies have been carried out in EC.[12–21] Chemotherapeutic agents have often been added to radiotherapy in the preoperative setting with the expectation of improved outcome. However, the addition of chemotherapy increases the toxicity of the treatment. Chemotherapy drugs most commonly used as radiosensitizers include fluoropyrimidines, taxanes, and platinum compounds.[22–25]

One of the first studies by Steiger and colleagues[26] combined 5-fluorouracil (5-FU) and mytomycin C or cisplatin with radiation therapy (50–60 Gy) in the preoperative setting in EC and observed a pathCR rate of 37% and a 2-year survival rate of 30%. Additional similar phase 2 trials followed, confirming the possible benefit to this therapeutic approach.[12–14] Subsequently, randomized trials evaluated the benefit of concurrent and sequential chemoradiation versus radiation alone (**Tables 1–3**), culminating in a prospective randomized phase 3 trial that documented the benefit of chemoradiation over radiation alone. In this study, conducted by the Radiation Therapy Oncology Group (RTOG),[17] 121 patients with EC

Table 1
Randomized trials of definitive chemoradiation versus radiotherapy

Study	Number of Patients	Histology	Treatment	Survival	Survival Difference (P)
Andersen et al,[50] 1984	82	SCC	RT (63 Gy) vs CT (Bleomycin) + RT (55 Gy)	2 y 11.9% 12%	.80
Araujo et al,[15] 1991	59	SCC	RT (50 Gy) vs CT (5-FU, MM, Bleomycin) + RT 50 Gy	5 y 6% 16%	NS
Cooper et al,[17] 1999	121	SCC/AC	RT 64 Gy vs CT (5-FU + CDDP) RT (50 Gy)	5 y 0% 26%	P<.001
Earle et al,[51] 1980	91	SCC	RT (50 or 60 Gy) vs CT (Bleomycin) + RT 50 Gy	5 y <8%	NS
Kaneta et al,[52] 1997	24	SCC	RT (60 Gy) CT (CDDP) + RT (60 Gy)	NR	NS
Li et al,[53] 2000	96	Ca	RT (60–70 Gy) CT (CDDP + 5-FU) + RT (5–60 Gy)	5 y 4.1% 28.8%	S
Roussel et al,[54] 1994	221	SCC	RT (40 Gy) CT (CDDP) + RT (40 Gy)	NR	P = .17
Slabber et al,[55] 1998	70	SCC	RT 40 Gy CT (CDDP + 5-FU) + RT (40 Gy)	NR	NS
Zhang,[56] 1984	99	SCC/AC	CT (Bleomycin 10 mg IM × 2-3/d + RT 39–73 Gy) RT 73 Gy		NS

Abbreviations: 5-FU, 5-Fluourouracil; AC, adenocarcinoma; CDDP, cisplatin; CT, chemotherapy; EB, external beam; HDBT, high-dose brachytherapy; IM, intramuscular; MM, mitomycin; MTX, methrotrexate; NR, nonreported; NS, nonsignificant; RT, radiation therapy; S, significant; SCC, squamous cell carcinoma.
Data from Refs.[15,17,50–56]

Table 2
Randomized trials of sequential chemoradiotherapy versus radiotherapy alone

Study	Number of Patients	Histology	Treatment	Survival	Survival Difference (P)
Hatlevoll et al,[57] 1992	100	SCC	RT (60 Gy) vs Sequential CT (CDDP) + RT	3 y 6% 0%	NS
Hishikawa et al,[58] 1991	62	SCC	RT (EB 60–70 Gy) or (EB 50–60 Gy + HDBT 10–15 Gy) CT fterafur PO + RT (EB or EB + HDRT)		NS
Roussel et al,[59] 1989	170	SCC	RT (56.25 Gy) Sequential CT (MTX) then RT 56.25 Gy	NR	NS
Wobbes et al,[60] 2001	221	SCC	RT (40 Gy (BED 45 Gy)) Sequential RT (40 Gy (BED 45 Gy)) then CT (CDDP)	2 y 15% 20%	P = .048
Zhou,[61] 1991	64	NR	RT (65–75 Gy) Sequential CT (CDDP + 5-FU++RT (65–75 Gy))	2 y 56.3% 34.6%	P = .05

Abbreviations: 5-FU, 5-Fluorouracil; CDDP, cisplatin; CT, chemotherapy; EB, external beam; Gy, gray; HDBT, high-dose brachytherapy; MTX, methrotrexate; NR, nonreported; NS, nonsignificant; PO, oral; RT, radiation therapy; SCC, squamous cell carcinoma.
Data from Refs.[57–61]

were randomized to concurrent chemotherapy and radiation versus radiation alone. In the chemoradiation arm, the total dose of radiation was 50 Gy in 25 fractions combined with 5-FU and cisplatin. In the radiation arm, the total dose was 64 Gy divided in 32 fractions. The interim analysis demonstrated improvement in overall survival in the chemoradiation arm; thus the randomization was stopped. The study remained open however, and additional patients were treated with

Table 3
Trials of definitive chemoradiation versus chemoradiation and surgery

Study	Number of Patients	Histology	Stage	Treatment	Survival	Survival Difference (P)
Bedenne et al,[20] 2007	259	SCC (90%) or AC	T3N0-1	CT (5-FU + Cisp × 2 cycles) + RT 46/23 Gy or 15/5 + 15/5 If response: Surgery or Further CRT (5-FU/CDDP × 3 cycles + RT 20/10 or 15/5)	2 y 34% 40%	NS
Stahl et al,[19] 2005	172	SCC	T3-4N0-1	CT (FLEP) + CT(PE) RT (40 Gy) + Surgery CT (FLEP) + CT(PE) RT (65 Gy)	3 y 64% 41%	NS

Abbreviations: 5-FU, 5-Fluorouracil; AC, adenocarcinoma; CDDP, cisplatin; CT, chemotherapy; FLEP, 5-Fluorouracil, leucovorin, etoposide, and cisplatin; NR, nonreported; NS, nonsignificant; RT, radiation therapy; SCC, squamous cell carcinoma.
Data from Stahl M, et al. Chemoradiation with and without surgery in patients with locally advanced squamous cell carcinoma of the esophagus. J Clin Oncol 2005;23:2310–7; and Bedenne L, et al. Chemoradiation followed by surgery compared with chemoradiation alone in squamous cancer of the esophagus: FFCD 9102. J Clin Oncol 2007;25:1160–8.

chemoradiation (while the radiation only arm was shut down). The 5-year overall survival for the chemoradiation arm was 26% (95% confidence interval [CI], 15%–37%) compared with 0% for the radiation arm. In the randomized portion of this study, 90% of the patients had squamous cell carcinoma, and in the nonrandomized portion, predominantly adenocarcinoma (with only 15% 5-year survival). The toxicity was significantly higher in the chemoradiation arm; acute toxicity grade 4 to 5 was 2% in the radiation arm compared to 10% in the chemoradiation arm. Recurrent local disease accounted for the majority of treatment failures.[17]

Based on the high local failure rate as well as a previous phase 2 study demonstrating that dose escalation to 64.8 Gy appeared to be well tolerated, dose-escalation in this context was examined. Specifically, the INT 0123 trial examined concurrent chemoradiation with cisplatin and 5-FU using either the standard dose (50.4 Gy) or an escalated dose (64.8 Gy).[18] A statistically insignificant detriment in survival was observed in the dose-escalated arm; however, it is worth noting that 7 of the 11 patient deaths in the dose-escalated arm occurred prior to the patient being treated with 50.4 Gy.

Further, not all trials of chemoradiation in this context have been positive. The Eastern Cooperative Oncology Group (ECOG) performed EST-1282, a randomized trial of preoperative radiation alone or in combination with 5-FU and mitomycin C in 119 patients with EC. After 40 Gy, the physician had the option for surgical evaluation or to continue with treatment with radiotherapy to an additional 20 Gy. The 5-year survival was not statistically significant (7% vs 9%).[16] However, despite EST-1282 being a negative trial, a review of 19 randomized trials by the Cochrane Library (including RTOG 85-01) showed that concurrent chemoradiotherapy provided a reduction in mortality with a hazard ratio (HR) of 0.73 (95% CI 0.64–0.84).[27]

In summary, most early trials demonstrated an advantage to the addition of chemotherapy to radiotherapy in the treatment of EC, as well as a lack of benefit from dose escalation.

Definitive Chemoradiation Versus Chemoradiation Plus Surgery

Two randomized studies have been performed comparing bimodality and trimodality therapy for esophageal cancer, with primary limitation being that both were performed only in patients with squamous cell histology (see **Table 2**). In the Fédération Francophone de Cancérologie

Digestive (FFCD) 9102 study, 444 patients received chemoradiotherapy with either 46 Gy in 4.5 weeks (2 Gy per fraction) or a split-course (2 × 15 Gy D1–5 and 22–26 at 3 Gy per fraction). This was followed by evaluation for objective response, with randomization of responders to either surgery or continuation of chemoradiation (3 cycles of 5FU-cisplatin).[20] Subsequent radiation was either continuous or as a split course to a total dose of 66 Gy or 45 Gy, respectively; however, the radiotherapy was amended to include only the conventional radiotherapy option (2 Gy per fraction). Following preoperative chemoradiation, 259 patients were randomized. The 2-year survival rate was similar for both groups, 34% in the chemoradiation only group versus 40% in trimodality group (adjusted odds ratio [OR] = 0.91; P = .56).[20] Unfortunately this study addresses the utility of bimodality therapy only in those patients who respond to chemoradiation. In addition, the alternate (split course) regimens of radiotherapy further confound the results.

An additional randomized trial in squamous cell carcinoma of the esophagus was performed by Stahl and colleagues,[19] who randomized 172 patients to induction chemotherapy followed by either chemoradiotherapy (40 Gy) followed by surgery, or additional chemoradiotherapy (at least 65 Gy) alone. The overall survival for both groups was similar (36% vs 39%), although surgery improved local tumor control. Worth noting is the excessive perioperative mortality (>12%) encountered in the surgery arms of both European trials, potentially negating any therapeutic benefit.

It is known from these trials and other studies that approximately 25% of patients achieve a pathCR[28–31] after preoperative chemoradiation. Because pathCR is associated with improved outcome, the benefit to surgical resection in this patient population is unclear. To partially address this question, RTOG 0246 evaluated definitive chemoradiation with a selective surgical salvage approach in patients with LEC. Patients received induction chemotherapy with 5-FU, cisplatin, and paclitaxel for 2 cycles, followed by concurrent chemoradiation with a total of 50.4 Gy in 28 fractions. Salvage esophagectomy was considered for patients with residual or recurrent EC without distant metastatic disease. The 1-year survival rate was 71% (95% CI <54%–82%), with an updated overall 5-year survival rate of 36.6% (95% CI, 22.3%–51.0%) at a median follow-up of 6.7 years.[21,32] However, only 12% of the entire population was alive long-term without surgery; thus it is unclear in whom surgical resection following chemoradiation can be safely omitted.

Positron Emission Tomography as a Predicting Tool

Positron emission tomography (PET) is currently part of initial staging in LEC, with the primary purpose to detect the occult metastases present in 15% to 20% of newly diagnosed patients.[33–36] PET is an assessment of glucose consumption by normal and abnormal tissues, performed by using 18-fluorodeoxyglucose (FDG). FDG is a radio-labeled metabolite whose uptake is associated with glycolysis and glucose transport. Tissue uptake of FDG is commonly reported by the standardized uptake value (SUV), which is a semiquantitative measure of the FDG uptake.[37] This value provides an indirect representation of cell proliferation, by quantitating cellular metabolic activity. Primary tumor SUV appears to correlate with patient outcome in EC in a variety of different contexts.

One of the first studies examining the use of PET for prognosis in EC determined baseline SUV max (iSUVmax) in patients undergoing primary surgery.[38] A high iSUVmax correlated with diminished survival, even in patients with early tumors and without nodal involvement. Later, PET was also studied as a predictor of histologic response after preoperative treatment. Several reports have found that SUV can be a prognosticator following preoperative chemotherapy or chemoradiation.[33,39–41] Suzuki and colleagues[37] reported on the iSUVmax in LEC patients undergoing definitive chemoradiation. The median iSUV was 12.7 (range 0–51). The higher the iSUVmax, the higher was the clinical stage and the lack of achievement of clinical complete response (clinCR). The estimated overall survival for patients with clinCR was 37.47 months and patients with less than clinCR were 12.6 months. Monjazeb and colleagues[42] also showed the PET complete response was a prognosticator of the outcome in patients who received bimodality therapy. Conversely, a German study found no correlation of post-treatment PET results with pathologic response or survival.[43] As PET response as a prognosticator of the outcome has conflicting results in the literature and has not been formally evaluated prospectively in a large group of patients, there is insufficient evidence to implement PET response in the clinic outside of a clinical trial.[44–46]

It is known that patients with pathCR have improved 5-year survival compared with patients with residual disease at esophagectomy (50% vs 22.6%).[47] In an attempt to improve upon PET response alone in determining response to therapy and generate a predictive model for pathCR in patients who have received concurrent chemoradiation for EC, the authors' group studied multiple clinical variables to determine their relationship to therapeutic response and pathCR.[48] The results of this study found that female sex, well or moderately differentiated histology, negative post-treatment biopsy, low postchemoradiation SUVmax, and baseline T stage were associated with pathCR. Unfortunately, none of these variables individually were able to predict pathCR with greater than 60% probability. This model is currently not applicable in the clinic, because a very small fraction of patients achieved a score above 160. This model may become relevant when the pathCR rate can be increased.

In the absence of a reliable pathCR model, the authors previously reported the association between clinCR and pathCR. Of 284 patients who completed trimodality therapy, 77% achieved clinCR; however, only 31% achieved pathCR. Thus clinicalCR has low specificity and therefore could not be used for clinical decision making for avoiding surgery.[49]

Based on previously mentined studies, PET might be used to identify subpopulations of patients with early stage disease or metabolic nonresponders after initial treatment who are more likely to be associated with poorer survival; therefore further therapy can be undertaken. However, much work remains to be done.

SUMMARY

Identifying patients with high probability of pathCR through predictive models that can incorporate clinical parameters and biomarkers is challenging and an area of active research. In the future, better understanding of the molecular biology involved in response should lead to rationally designed clinical trials targeting those patients who are at risk for treatment failure.

REFERENCES

1. Ferlay J, Shin HR, Bray F, et al. Estimates of worldwide burden of cancer in 2008: GLOBOCAN 2008. Int J Cancer 2010;127:2893–917.
2. Jemal A, Center MM, DeSantis C, et al. Global patterns of cancer incidence and mortality rates and trends. Cancer Epidemiol Biomarkers Prev 2010; 19:1893–907.
3. Pearson JG. The present status and future potential of radiotherapy in the management of esophageal cancer. Cancer 1977;39:882–90.
4. Van Hagen P, Hulshof MC, van Lanschot JJ, et al. Preoperative chemoradiotherapy for esophageal or junctional cancer. N Engl J Med 2012;366: 2074–84.

5. Gholipour C, Shalchi RA, Abbasi M. A histopathological study of esophageal cancer on the western side of the Caspian littoral from 1994 to 2003. Dis Esophagus 2008;21:322–7.

6. Tran GD, Sun XD, Abnet CC, et al. Prospective study of risk factors for esophageal and gastric cancers in the Linxian general population trial cohort in China. Int J Cancer 2005;113:456–63.

7. Pohl H, Welch HG. The role of overdiagnosis and reclassification in the marked increase of esophageal adenocarcinoma incidence. J Natl Cancer Inst 2005;97:142–6.

8. Brown LM, Devesa SS, Chow WH. Incidence of adenocarcinoma of the esophagus among white Americans by sex, stage, and age. J Natl Cancer Inst 2008;100:1184–7.

9. Rice TW, Rusch VW, Ishwaran H, et al. Cancer of the esophagus and esophagogastric junction: data-driven staging for the seventh edition of the American Joint Committee on Cancer/International Union Against Cancer Cancer Staging Manuals. Cancer 2010;116:3763–73.

10. Rice TW, Rusch VW, Apperson-Hansen C, et al. Worldwide esophageal cancer collaboration. Dis Esophagus 2009;22:1–8.

11. Nigro ND, Vaitkevicius VK, Considine B Jr. Combined therapy for cancer of the anal canal: a preliminary report. 1974. Dis Colon Rectum 1993;36:709–11.

12. John MJ, Flam MS, Mowry PA, et al. Radiotherapy alone and chemoradiation for nonmetastatic esophageal carcinoma. A critical review of chemoradiation. Cancer 1989;63:2397–403.

13. Keane TJ, Harwood AR, Elhakim T, et al. Radical radiation therapy with 5-fluorouracil infusion and mitomycin C for oesophageal squamous carcinoma. Radiother Oncol 1985;4:205–10.

14. Herskovic A, Leichman L, Lattin P, et al. Chemo/radiation with and without surgery in the thoracic esophagus: the Wayne State experience. Int J Radiat Oncol Biol Phys 1988;15:655–62.

15. Araújo CM, Souhami L, Gil RA, et al. A randomized trial comparing radiation therapy versus concomitant radiation therapy and chemotherapy in carcinoma of the thoracic esophagus. Cancer 1991;67:2258–61.

16. Smith TJ, Ryan LM, Douglass HO Jr, et al. Combined chemoradiotherapy vs. radiotherapy alone for early stage squamous cell carcinoma of the esophagus: a study of the Eastern Cooperative Oncology Group. Int J Radiat Oncol Biol Phys 1998;42:269–76.

17. Cooper JS, Guo MD, Herskovic A, et al. Chemoradiotherapy of locally advanced esophageal cancer: long-term follow-up of a prospective randomized trial (RTOG 85-01). Radiation Therapy Oncology Group. JAMA 1999;281:1623–7.

18. Minsky BD, Pajak TF, Ginsberg RJ, et al. INT 0123 (Radiation Therapy Oncology Group 94-05) phase III trial of combined-modality therapy for esophageal cancer: high-dose versus standard-dose radiation therapy. J Clin Oncol 2002;20:1167–74.

19. Stahl M, Stuschke M, Lehmann N, et al. Chemoradiation with and without surgery in patients with locally advanced squamous cell carcinoma of the esophagus. J Clin Oncol 2005;23:2310–7.

20. Bedenne L, Michel P, Bouché O, et al. Chemoradiation followed by surgery compared with chemoradiation alone in squamous cancer of the esophagus: FFCD 9102. J Clin Oncol 2007;25:1160–8.

21. Swisher SG, Winter KA, Komaki RU, et al. A Phase II study of a paclitaxel-based chemoradiation regimen with selective surgical salvage for resectable locoregionally advanced esophageal cancer: initial reporting of RTOG 0246. Int J Radiat Oncol Biol Phys 2012;82:1967–72.

22. Byfield JE, Calabro-Jones P, Klisak I, et al. Pharmacologic requirements for obtaining sensitization of human tumor cells in vitro to combined 5-Fluorouracil or ftorafur and X rays. Int J Radiat Oncol Biol Phys 1982;8:1923–33.

23. Byfield JE. 5-Fluorouracil radiation sensitization–a brief review. Invest New Drugs 1989;7:111–6.

24. Dewit L. Combined treatment of radiation and cis-diamminedichloroplatinum (II): a review of experimental and clinical data. Int J Radiat Oncol Biol Phys 1987;13:403–26.

25. Creane M, Seymour CB, Colucci S, et al. Radiobiological effects of docetaxel (Taxotere): a potential radiation sensitizer. Int J Radiat Biol 1999;75:731–7.

26. Steiger Z, Franklin R, Wilson RF, et al. Complete eradication of squamous cell carcinoma of the esophagus with combined chemotherapy and radiotherapy. Am Surg 1981;47:95–8.

27. Wong R, Malthaner R. Combined chemotherapy and radiotherapy (without surgery) compared with radiotherapy alone in localized carcinoma of the esophagus. Cochrane Database Syst Rev 2006:CD002092.

28. Rohatgi P, Swisher SG, Correa AM, et al. Characterization of pathologic complete response after preoperative chemoradiotherapy in carcinoma of the esophagus and outcome after pathologic complete response. Cancer 2005;104:2365–72.

29. Chirieac LR, Swisher SG, Ajani JA, et al. Posttherapy pathologic stage predicts survival in patients with esophageal carcinoma receiving preoperative chemoradiation. Cancer 2005;103:1347–55.

30. Berger AC, Farma J, Scott WJ, et al. Complete response to neoadjuvant chemoradiotherapy in esophageal carcinoma is associated with significantly improved survival. J Clin Oncol 2005;23:4330–7.

31. Donahue JM, Nichols FC, Li Z, et al. Complete pathologic response after neoadjuvant chemoradiotherapy for esophageal cancer is associated with enhanced survival. Ann Thorac Surg 2009; 87:392–8 [discussion: 398–9].

32. Swisher S, Moughan J, Komaki R, et al. Final results of RTOG 0246: a phase II study of selective surgical resection for locoregionally advanced esophageal cancer treated with a paclitaxel-based chemoradiation regimen [abstract]. J Clin Oncol 2012;30(Suppl 34).

33. Downey RJ, Akhurst T, Ilson D, et al. Whole body 18FDG-PET and the response of esophageal cancer to induction therapy: results of a prospective trial. J Clin Oncol 2003;21:428–32.

34. Flamen P, Lerut A, Van Cutsem E, et al. Utility of positron emission tomography for the staging of patients with potentially operable esophageal carcinoma. J Clin Oncol 2000;18:3202–10.

35. Heeren PA, Jager PL, Bongaerts F, et al. Detection of distant metastases in esophageal cancer with (18)F-FDG PET. J Nucl Med 2004;45:980–7.

36. Kato H, Nakajima M, Sohda M, et al. The clinical application of (18)F-fluorodeoxyglucose positron emission tomography to predict survival in patients with operable esophageal cancer. Cancer 2009; 115:3196–203.

37. Suzuki A, Xiao L, Hayashi Y, et al. Prognostic significance of baseline positron emission tomography and importance of clinical complete response in patients with esophageal or gastroesophageal junction cancer treated with definitive chemoradiotherapy. Cancer 2011;117:4823–33.

38. Rizk N, Downey RJ, Akhurst T, et al. Preoperative 18[F]-fluorodeoxyglucose positron emission tomography standardized uptake values predict survival after esophageal adenocarcinoma resection. Ann Thorac Surg 2006;81:1076–81.

39. Weber WA, Ott K, Becker K, et al. Prediction of response to preoperative chemotherapy in adenocarcinomas of the esophagogastric junction by metabolic imaging. J Clin Oncol 2001;19:3058–65.

40. Flamen P, Van Cutsem E, Lerut A, et al. Positron emission tomography for assessment of the response to induction radiochemotherapy in locally advanced oesophageal cancer. Ann Oncol 2002; 13:361–8.

41. Skinner HD, McCurdy MR, Echeverria AE, et al. Metformin use and improved response to therapy in esophageal adenocarcinoma. Acta Oncol 2013;52:1002–9.

42. Monjazeb AM, Riedlinger G, Aklilu M, et al. Outcomes of patients with esophageal cancer staged with [18F]fluorodeoxyglucose positron emission tomography (FDG-PET): can postchemoradiotherapy FDG-PET predict the utility of resection? J Clin Oncol 2010;28:4714–21.

43. Vallböhmer D, Hölscher AH, Dietlein M, et al. [18F]-Fluorodeoxyglucose-positron emission tomography for the assessment of histopathologic response and prognosis after completion of neoadjuvant chemoradiation in esophageal cancer. Ann Surg 2009;250:888–94.

44. Ilson DH, Minsky BD, Ku GY, et al. Phase 2 trial of induction and concurrent chemoradiotherapy with weekly irinotecan and cisplatin followed by surgery for esophageal cancer. Cancer 2012;118:2820–7.

45. Kauppi JT, Oksala N, Salo JA, et al. Locally advanced esophageal adenocarcinoma: response to neoadjuvant chemotherapy and survival predicted by ([18F])FDG-PET/CT. Acta Oncol 2012; 51:636–44.

46. Klaeser B, Nitzsche E, Schuller JC, et al. Limited predictive value of FDG-PET for response assessment in the preoperative treatment of esophageal cancer: results of a prospective multi-center trial (SAKK 75/02). Onkologie 2009;32:724–30.

47. Scheer RV, Fakiris AJ, Johnstone PA. Quantifying the benefit of a pathologic complete response after neoadjuvant chemoradiotherapy in the treatment of esophageal cancer. Int J Radiat Oncol Biol Phys 2011;80:996–1001.

48. Ajani JA, Correa AM, Hofstetter WL, et al. Clinical parameters model for predicting pathologic complete response following preoperative chemoradiation in patients with esophageal cancer. Ann Oncol 2012;23:2638–42.

49. Cheedella NK, Suzuki A, Xiao L, et al. Association between clinical complete response and pathological complete response after preoperative chemoradiation in patients with gastroesophageal cancer: analysis in a large cohort. Ann Oncol 2013;24(5):1262–6.

50. Andersen AP, Berdal P, Edsmyr F, et al. Irradiation, chemotherapy and surgery in esophageal cancer: a randomized clinical study. The first Scandinavian trial in esophageal cancer. Radiother Oncol 1984;2: 179–88.

51. Earle JD, Gelber RD, Moertel CG, et al. A controlled evaluation of combined radiation and bleomycin therapy for squamous cell carcinoma of the esophagus. Int J Radiat Oncol Biol Phys 1980;6:821–6.

52. Kaneta T, Takai Y, Nemoto K, et al. Effects of combination chemoradiotherapy with daily low-dose CDDP for esophageal cancer–results of a randomized trial. Gan To Kagaku Ryoho 1997;24:2099–104 [in Japanese].

53. Li A, Su B, Lin Y. 48 Patients with advanced esophageal cancer treated with DDP+5-Fu combined radiotherapy. Chinese Journal Clinical Oncology Rehabilitation 2000;7(6):79–80.

54. Roussel A, Haegele P, Paillot B. Results of the EORTC-GTCCT Phase III trial of irradiation vs

irradiation and CDDP in inoperable esophageal cancer. Proc Annu Meet Am Soc Clin Oncol 1994; 13:199.

55. Slabber CF, Nel JS, Schoeman L, et al. A randomized study of radiotherapy alone versus radiotherapy plus 5-fluorouracil and platinum in patients with inoperable, locally advanced squamous cancer of the esophagus. Am J Clin Oncol 1984;21:462–5.

56. Zhang ZF. Radiation combined with bleomycin in esophageal carcinoma–a randomized study of 99 patients. Zhonghua Zhong Liu Za Zhi 1984;6:372–4 [in Chinese].

57. Hatlevoll R, Hagen S, Hansen HS, et al. Bleomycin/cis-platin as neoadjuvant chemotherapy before radical radiotherapy in localized, inoperable carcinoma of the esophagus. A prospective randomized multicentre study: the second Scandinavian trial in esophageal cancer. Radiother Oncol 1992;24:114–6.

58. Hishikawa Y, Miura T, Oshitani T, et al. A randomized prospective study of adjuvant chemotherapy after radiotherapy in unresectable esophageal carcinoma. Dis Esophagus 1991;4(2):85–90.

59. Roussel A, Bleiberg H, Dalesio O, et al. Palliative therapy of inoperable oesophageal carcinoma with radiotherapy and methotrexate: final results of a controlled clinical trial. Int J Radiat Oncol Biol Phys 1989;16:67–72.

60. Wobbes T, Baron B, Paillot B, et al. Prospective randomised study of split-course radiotherapy versus cisplatin plus split-course radiotherapy in inoperable squamous cell carcinoma of the oesophagus. Eur J Cancer 2001;37:470–7.

61. Zhou JC. Randomized trial of combined chemotherapy including high dose cisplatin and radiotherapy for esophageal cancer. Zhonghua Zhong Liu Za Zhi 1991;13:291–4 [in Chinese].

Salvage Esophagectomy in the Management of Recurrent or Persistent Esophageal Carcinoma

Jenifer Marks, MD[a], David C. Rice, MD[b],
Stephen G. Swisher, MD[b,*]

KEYWORDS

- Esophagectomy • Salvage • Adenocarcinoma • Squamous • Chemotherapy • Radiation

KEY POINTS

- Salvage esophagectomy is a viable treatment option in the management of recurrent or persistent esophageal cancer (EC) and can be performed with acceptable morbidity and mortality in a select group of patients.
- Patient selection should include a complete restaging evaluation, cardiopulmonary testing, and an assessment of functional status. The majority of patients with persistent or recurrent EC are not candidates for salvage resection.
- Operative considerations the authors have adopted for salvage esophagectomy include
  - Proper conduit choice and the use of alternative conduits, if necessary
  - Staging the resection and reconstruction in high-risk patients
  - Using an omental tissue transposition to protect the anastomosis
  - Review preoperative radiation treatment records and if at all possible perform the anastomosis out of the previous field.
- The authors have shown that carefully selected patients undergoing a salvage resection have outcomes similar to those undergoing a planned esophagectomy after induction chemoradiotherapy.

 Video of salvage esophagectomy with omental transfer accompanies this article at http://www.thoracic.theclinics.com/

INTRODUCTION

The optimal treatment of locally advanced EC is controversial. There are patient, tumor, and oncologist preferences that influence treatment decisions. Patient factors include a previous history of cancer, major comorbidities, previous abdominal operations, and performance status (PS).

Additional tumor factors include location in the esophagus, histology, tumor length, and the depth of invasion through the esophageal wall. A large majority of upper esophageal squamous cell cancers (SCCs) throughout the world are treated with definitve chemoradiotherapy (dCRT). It has been established that surgical resection immediately after chemoradiotherapy (CRT) does not

a Division of Thoracic Surgery, Hackensack University Medical Center, 30 Prospect Avenue, Hackensack, NJ, USA; b Department of Thoracic and Cardiovascular Surgery, The University of Texas, MD Anderson Cancer Center, T. Boone Pickens Academic Tower (FCT19.5048), 1515 Holcombe Boulevard, Unit 1489, Houston, TX 77030, USA
* Corresponding author.
E-mail address: sswisher@mdanderson.org

Thorac Surg Clin 23 (2013) 559–567
http://dx.doi.org/10.1016/j.thorsurg.2013.08.001
1547-4127/13/$ – see front matter © 2013 Elsevier Inc. All rights reserved.

change the overall survival in this group of patients.[1,2] These patients may be offered salvage resection, however, if they have gross persistent disease after completion of dCRT or recurrent disease in the future. Outcomes of salvage resection for upper esophageal SCC are well described in the literature.[3–6]

Such a consensus on the optimal treatment of patients with lower-third esophageal adenocarcinoma does not exist. Most centers offer multimodality therapy for fit patients with a lower-third locally advanced esophageal adenocarcinoma, which may consist of induction CRT followed by resection, induction chemotherapy followed by resection, or dCRT alone. Patients receiving dCRT alone for either upper esophageal SCC or mid- to lower esophageal adenocarcinoma have a 20% to 60% local recurrence rate and may need further means of local control. Salvage esophagectomy is also an option in a select group of patients with local/regional recurrent adenocarcinoma after dCRT.

The definition of salvage esophagectomy is not consistent within the literature. Some investigators have used greater than 90 days from completion of dCRT as a time determination after which the resection is considered salvage. Others have used intent to treat as the determining factor; thus, a salvage resection is any resection that was not part of the initial treatment plan irrespective of when it occurs after dCRT. The population of patients with EC that present for resection after completing other types of therapy is diverse; hence, it becomes difficult to have an all-encompassing definition of salvage esophagectomy. Important factors to remember in defining salvage resection and its outcomes are that these patients have received definitive doses of radiation and chemotherapy prior to presentation for resection and careful patient selection and how the operation is performed are key to its success as a viable treatment option.

An overwhelming majority of the data on outcomes after salvage esophagectomy describe patients with local recurrence after dCRT for esophageal SCC. Salvage resection in this setting has been shown associated with a significantly higher morbidity and mortality than elective esophagectomy.[4–7] The authors' recently published data, however, suggest the overall risk of salvage resection for patients with recurrent or persistent esophageal adenocarcinoma may not be increased compared with that of patients matched on 11 preoperative patient and tumor characteristics undergoing a planned resection after induction CRT[8]; 65 patients undergoing salvage resection were compared with matched patients undergoing planned resection after CRT and there were no significant differences in the overall morbidity and mortality in this study. Outcomes in the current study are improved over those of the initial report of salvage esophagectomy from the authors' institution.[9] The authors' approach and several technical points thought to contribute to improved outcomes are discussed.

Many patients with recurrent EC after dCRT are not candidates for salvage resection due to poor PS or distant disease. As discussed later, a detailed preoperative physiologic evaluation and complete restaging should be performed. Patients with a good PS and no evidence of distant disease after a complete restaging evaluation are those in whom a salvage resection is potentially beneficial. Additional preoperative planning may be required in terms of conduit choice depending on the location of the tumor and the original radiation fields.

RELEVANT ANATOMY

Recurrent squamous cell ECs of the upper and midesophagus can involve the larynx, trachea, recurrent laryngeal or vagus nerves, and other surrounding soft tissues in the neck. Resection after dCRT may be difficult due to adherent tissue planes and local tumor effect. Careful evaluation of the vocal cords and airway should be performed preoperatively in addition to detailed endoscopic examination of the lesion to be resected. Tracheal invasion is generally considered a contraindication to salvage resection. Tracheal resection with primary anastomosis or construction of a mediastinal tracheostomy may be considered under highly select circumstances at specialized centers but generally is not offered. Proximal and distal margins should be estimated preoperatively with detailed imaging and endoscopy and plans made with supportive services if a laryngeal resection is thought necessary. If an R0 resection cannot be obtained, no resection should be offered.

Reconstruction after resection for upper esophageal SCC is performed most often with a gastric conduit. The entire length of the stomach can be tubularized and brought up to the neck because the proximal greater curvature has usually not been radiated in this setting. If prior gastric surgery has been performed for other reasons, then the colon or jejunum may be used for reconstruction.[10,11]

Recurrent disease in the distal esophagus usually poses less of an anatomic challenge if a tumor is confined to the esophagus. Invasion of the aorta or spine precludes resection, but most often a margin is obtained around the primary tumor without taking additional major structures. Portions of the liver or diaphragm are resected en bloc with the lesion if an R0 resection is obtained. Careful attention should be paid to the distal aspect of the lesion if it extends into the stomach because adequate margins may compromise the final conduit length. Radiation fields should also be reviewed because full-dose radiation to the cardia may render the stomach unsuitable for conduit formation. Again, alternative conduits, such as the colon or a long-segment jejunal interposition, may be necessary and should be anticipated and planned for preoperatively.[10,11]

CLINICAL PRESENTATION

Patients with recurrent disease after dCRT may present with symptoms of the primary tumor or they may be completely asymptomatic. Recurrences are often picked up on surveillance endoscopy or imaging before any symptoms have developed. Other patients may experience symptoms similar to those of their original lesion, such as dysphagia, hoarseness, weight loss, chest pain, cough, and gastrointestinal bleeding.

Complicated presentations, such as esophageal perforation, tracheoesophageal fistula (TEF), or aortoesophageal fistula, are less common but do occur. Symptoms of a perforation or TEF may include persistent fever, cough, aspiration pneumonia, or mediastinal sepsis. As discussed previously, tracheal involvement generally precludes offering a salvage resection except in select situations. If the esophageal perforation does not involve a fistula, however, and patients are shown free of distant disease, there are several options, one of which is to offer patients a staged procedure. This option is discussed later, but initial diversion, if less-invasive means such as stent placement have failed, followed by staged reconstruction allows treatment of the perforation, time for recovery, and surgical treatment of the cancer.

An aortoesophageal fistula may present with mild or massive hematemesis, anemia, or gastrointestinal bleeding. Classically it has been described as presenting with Chiari triad, which includes midthoracic chest pain, a sentinel arterial hemorrhage, and final exsanguination hours to months after an asymptomatic interval. Several case reports describe this presentation in association with EC although it is found most often in association with thoracic aortic aneurysms.[12,13] Emergency procedures, such as an aortic stent graft, may control the acute bleeding but they are purely palliative. Generally an esophageal stent should not be placed if an aortic stent has been placed, because the 2 rubbing against one another is likely to worsen the situation, although short-term survival with this technique has been

reported.[14] These patients are not candidates for salvage resection and palliative measures should be taken to facilitate patient comfort.

DIAGNOSIS AND CLINICAL RESTAGING

The diagnosis of recurrent or persistent EC is made most often from biopsies taken during endoscopy. CT or PET imaging may reveal a mass but this should always be confirmed histologically with a biopsy. In addition to histologic confirmation of cancer, documentation of tumor length, location of the gastroesophageal junction and its relation to the tumor, involvement of the cardia, and the presence or absence of Barrett's esophagus should all be documented in detail. Endoscopic ultrasound should be performed to evaluate the depth of invasion in the esophageal wall for presence of suspicious lymph nodes and to rule out aortic or tracheal invasion. For tumors in the upper and midesophagus, broncoscopy should be performed to evaluate for tracheal invasion or any evidence of a TEF.

In addition to esophagogastroduodenoscopy/ endoscopic ultrasound, a CT/PET should be performed to evaluate for distant disease. Distant lymph node involvement, such as a supraclavicular or high paratracheal node in association with a gastroesophageal junction adenocarcinoma, is not a contraindication to performing resection, but involvement suggests a systemic process and the implications of distant nodal disease should be discussed fully with patients prior to proceeding. Retroperitoneal nodes below the celiac vessels and low periaortic or paracaval nodes are generally considered distant disease and, if proved to be malignant, a resection is not offered.

PATIENT SELECTION

Patient selection is one of the most important factors in determining the outcomes after salvage esophagectomy. Many patients who receive dCRT as initial treatment have poor PS and are not good surgical candidates at the time of the original diagnosis. Of those patients with persistent disease after dCRT, a select subgroup has the PS to withstand salvage resection. Others have progression or distant disease and are not candidates for resection. Those with borderline decreased PS may be allowed additional time for recovery and nutritional repletion followed by re-evaluation at a later date.

Preoperative physiologic and pulmonary testing should be performed as is routine prior to any esophagectomy. Complete pulmonary function tests and a cardiac evaluation based on individual risk factors provide valuable information in deciding to which patients to offer salvage resection. Patient compliance and participation in postoperative pulmonary toilet, ambulation, and physical therapy are important factors in minimizing the morbidity associated with any esophagectomy. The authors have shown that careful selection of patients who are medically fit with local disease only achieve outcomes similar to those of patients undergoing planned esophagectomy after induction CRT.[8] Morita and colleagues[4] have also published extensively on salvage esophagectomy and report improved outcomes in the most recent series after adopting stricter surgical indications.

A select group of patients presenting with esophageal perforation can be managed with a 2-stage approach if they meet the other criteria for resection (ie, medically fit with no distant disease and no fistula to either the trachea or aorta). Initially, as with any esophageal perforation, the contamination and sepsis need to be controlled and treated with antibiotics. An esophageal stent may be placed over the perforation and time allowed for resuscitation. Patients should be evaluated for distant disease and, if none is demonstrated, resection, diversion, and jejunostomy can be performed as the first of a 2-stage salvage procedure (**Fig. 1**). These procedures are done during the initial hospitalization for the perforation if patients are fit or after a period of time during which the stent has sealed the perforation and when patients are allowed to recover and prepare for resection and diversion. Reconstruction is then performed after a period of 6 to 12 weeks during which patients are again staged and offered resection only if an R0 resection is achieved and there is no distant disease.

Not all patients with EC who present with an acute perforation are candidates for such an approach, but the authors encourage careful evaluation of the overall oncologic picture when faced with this situation because some patients are able to undergo a 2-stage salvage resection with curative intent despite presenting with a perforation.

Operative Planning

In addition to restaging all patients who present for salvage resection, all available imaging and endoscopic reports from the time of initial diagnosis should be reviewed. Detailed review of the proximal and distal extent of the original lesion and any involved nodes is essential in planning the resection and reconstruction. Consultation with head and neck oncologic surgeons may be necessary if a tumor is higher than approximately 15 cm.

Radiation records should be obtained and reviewed to determine if the recurrence is an infield or out-of-field recurrence, because this may necessitate further therapy after resection. The extent of the cardia and proximal stomach that received full-dose radiation should also be reviewed carefully because this may alter plans for reconstruction. A greater curvature that has received full-dose radiation may not be the ideal site for the anastomosis or even a viable conduit for this procedure. Dose and the extent of esophageal irradiation should also be noted and, whenever possible, the anastomosis performed in an area of esophagus that has not been radiated.

Conduit Selection

Many salvage resections are performed using the stomach as the conduit; however, some require alternate choices and additional preoperative imaging. Previous mediastinal or neck radiation, tumor length, previous thoracic or abdominal operations, and major comorbidities that may affect the stomach (ie, gastroparesis or gastric outlet obstruction from diabetes or peptic ulcer disease) are all factors to consider when choosing an organ for conduit creation. If the colon is used for reconstruction, a CT angiogram of the abdomen and pelvis is usually of sufficient quality to confirm appropriate blood supply for a transposition. Diseases of the mesentery or other abdominal organs may affect the mobilization and lie of the conduit and should also be evaluated on preoperative imaging. Additionally, colonoscopy or barium enema should be obtained to rule out any intrinsic luminal pathology. Reconstruction with a colon conduit is well described in the literature and is not described further.

Long-segment supercharged jejunal graft

A long-segment jejunal pedicle with microvascular augmentation is the conduit of choice most often used at the authors' institution if the stomach is not available. The reconstruction is performed with a plastic surgery team and both the technique and outcomes of this operation are published.[10,11] A long-segment of pedicled jejunum is mobilized in the abdomen with its vascular pedicle and most often passed through the retrosternal route to then anastomose with the proximal esophagus in the neck. The vascular supply of the jejunal pedicle is based off the third or fourth jejunal branch of the superior mesenteric artery whereas a more proximal branch is divided during mobilization and serves as the vessel for microvascular anastomosis to the mammary vessels.

Supercharging of the jejunal pedicle in this manner allows additional arterial inflow and venous drainage to help alleviate the venous congestion

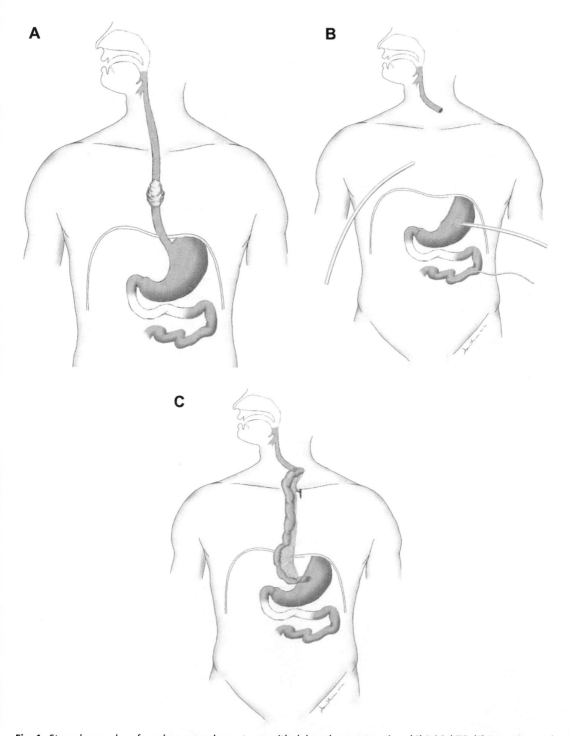

Fig. 1. Staged procedure for salvage esophagectomy with delayed reconstruction. (*A*) Initial EC. (*B*) Resection and diversion. (*C*) Reconstruction with supercharged jejunum.

that often occurs. Additional graft length can be obtained through this method so that high cervical-enteric anastomoses are made, if necessary. The retrosternal route keeps the conduit out of the posterior mediastinum, which is important if additional radiation is considered for the primary tumor bed or if the posterior mediastinum is hostile from prior interventions.

In addition to the choice of conduit, careful handling of and preservation of the conduit is essential. The conduit should be passed gently through the hiatus into the posterior mediastinum or retrosternal space, taking care not to twist the vascular pedicle. If the retrosternal route is used, it should be of ample size to accommodate the conduit without compression of the conduit itself or the vascular supply. When using this route, the authors routinely resect a portion of the manubrium, clavicular head, and, if necessary, the medial portion of the first rib to allow space in the thoracic inlet for the conduit to lie. Bony compression and stricture or scarring in this area can be a problem if the thoracic inlet is not large enough to easily accommodate the conduit and its mesentery.

Two-Staged Procedure

Staging the resection and reconstruction is another option in the salvage setting to help decrease potential morbidity (see **Fig. 1**). As discussed for patients presenting with isolated esophageal perforation, the morbidity associated with a resection and diversion is less than that of full reconstruction and may serve as a litmus test for both patients and the biology of the tumor.[15,16] Resection alone is a shorter operation with less risk to patients because there is no anastomosis. If patients are able to tolerate the resection, regain adequate function status, and remain nutritionally replete, then restaging is again undertaken. If there is no sign of distant disease or local progression that precludes an R0 resection on restaging studies, then reconstruction can be performed.

The possibility of disease progression after diversion and no ultimate reconstruction is discussed with patients and families from the beginning so they are aware that the esophagostomy is potentially permanent if their disease progresses. Again, these patients are presenting in a condition that requires diversion and, as such, options are limited but this approach maintains the possibility of a curative resection in the absence of distant disease. The 2-staged approach has been shown to have acceptable morbidity and mortality and should be considered if the reconstruction is complex and lengthy.[16]

Omental Tissue Transposition

Omental tissue transposition into the chest is another technique that may decrease the morbidity associated with a salvage esophagectomy.[17,18] Based on 2 or 3 major feeding vessels from the right gastroepiploic artery, a pedicle of omentum may be mobilized into the chest along with the gastric conduit to wrap the anastomosis. This augmentation to a standard anastomosis has been described by several investigators and the data suggest that the incidence and perhaps severity of anastomotic leaks are reduced (**Fig. 2**).[17–19] The omentum can also be placed in between the anastomosis and the trachea or aorta to potentially contain and limit associated organ injury (ie, fistula) if a leak does occur (see **Fig. 2**C, Video 1).

CLINICAL OUTCOMES

Previous reports of outcomes after salvage esophagectomy have been notable for high morbidity and mortality, which have limited acceptance of the procedure (**Table 1**).[4–7] As discussed previously, a majority of these reports describe

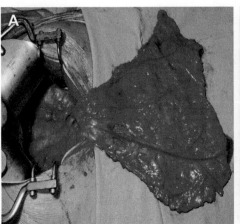
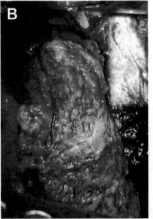
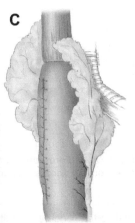

Fig. 2. Omental tissue transposition. (*A*) Preservation of 2 to 3 vessels supplying the omental pedicle. (*B*) Omental pedicle wrapped around conduit in chest. (*C*) Schematic of pedicle interposition between anastomosis and trachea.

Table 1
Recent reports of salvage esophagectomy outcomes

| | Gardner-Thorpe et al,[5] 2007 | Morita et al,[a,4] 2011 | | Marks et al,[8] 2012 | |
	All Salvage	Planned	Salvage	Planned	Salvage
# Patients	109	197	27	521	65
Leak (%)	6–38	23	37	11	19
Conduit necrosis (%)	0–25	NR	NR	1	5
Hospital mortality (%)	6–33	2	7	3	5
Survival					
Median (mo)	7–32	NR	NR	48	32
5-y Overall (%)	0–35[b]	41	51	45	32

Abbreviation: NR, not reported.
[a] Study included 3 groups of patients, only 2 of which are relevant for comparison in this setting.
[b] Survival reported for those studies in the analysis with the reported data.
Data from Refs.[4,5,8]

resection in patients with recurrent upper esophageal squamous cell carcinoma. A review by Gardner-Thorpe and colleagues[5] summarizes 9 other published series of salvage esophagectomy, totaling 105 patients, 9 of whom had adenocarcinoma. Rates of pneumonia (0%–38%), anastomotic leak (6%–38%), and conduit loss (8%–25%) were higher than what is expected after an elective esophagectomy. Also included in the table are 2 other recent series, one from the authors' institution, which describe outcomes in salvage patients compared with those of patients undergoing a planned resection after induction CRT.

The authors' data suggest that patients presenting for salvage resection with distal esophageal adenocarcinoma are in general a higher risk group of patients with more comorbidities than those offered trimodality therapy initially.[8] Matched-pair analysis demonstrates that when matched on 11 preoperative patient and tumor characteristics, salvage resection can be performed with the same morbidity and mortality as a planned resection after induction CRT. The incidence of major pulmonary event, anastomotic leak, and conduit necrosis was no different between the 2 groups. In addition, the authors have chosen to report all anastomotic leaks, grades I to IV, in their series (**Table 2**). The majority of the literature regarding anastomotic leak, including the 2 other series outlined in **Table 1**, does not define the grade of the leak reported. There is a trend to only report leaks requiring a return to the operating room in the literature. Grades I and II leaks do not require surgical intervention; however, they are still leaks and should be reported as such. If only leaks requiring surgical intervention were reported, the authors' leak rate in the salvage group would be only 10%, well within the range expected after elective esophagectomy after CRT.

Several reasons explain the outcome differences in the authors' series compared with those in the remainder of the literature. The authors'

Table 2
Grading of anastomotic leak

| | Morita et al,[4] 2011 | | Marks et al,[8] 2012 | |
	Planned (%)	Salvage (%)	Planned (%)	Salvage (%)
Anastomotic leak	23	37	11	19
Grade I: radiographic only	NR	NR	4	2
Grade II: minor intervention	NR	NR	3	6
Grade III: surgical repair	NR	NR	3	6
Grade IV: conduit loss	NR	NR	1	5

Abbreviation: NR, not reported.
Data from Morita M, Kumashiro R, Hisamatsu Y, et al. Clinical significance of salvage esophagectomy for remnant or recurrent cancer following definitive chemoradiotherapy. J Gastroenterol 2011;46:1284–91; and Marks J, Hofstetter W, Correa A, et al. Salvage esophagectomy after failed definitive chemoradiation for esophageal adenocarcinoma. Ann Thorac Surg 2012;94(4):1126–33.

series describes patients with mid- to lower esophageal adenocarcinoma only, a distinct and separate group of patients than those with upper esophageal SCC. Although CRT regimens may or may not be similar for the 2 disease sites, the proximity of the cervical esophagus to other critical structures in the neck potentially complicates and adds to the morbidity of salvage resections for SCC. Anastomosis within the radiated field is often unavoidable, although undesirable, in more proximal tumors undergoing salvage resection. The recent Morita and colleagues[4] article, however, also describes improved outcomes after salvage resection in patients with mostly squamous cell EC compared with the earlier literature. This is further evidence that salvage resection can be performed with acceptable morbidity and mortality and should be offered to a select group of patients with persistent or recurrent disease after CRT.

The authors have adopted the management and technical points described previously and believe they are critical for improved outcomes:

1. Strict patient selection based on PS and complete restaging
2. Proper conduit choice and creation with the use of alternative conduits if necessary
3. Staging the procedure in high-risk patients
4. Omental tissue transposition into the chest to protect the anastomosis
5. When possible, performing the anastomosis out of the previous radiation field

Additionally, the planning, implementation, and compliance with fast-track postoperative care pathways have contributed to the lower overall morbidity seen in current series describing esophagectomy outcomes.[8,20]

SUMMARY

Salvage esophagectomy is a viable treatment option in the management of recurrent or persistent EC. Preoperative evaluations, including complete restaging to confirm the absence of distant metastatic disease, cardiopulmonary physiologic testing, and assessment of PS, are key to identifying the group of patients in whom a salvage resection can be performed with acceptable morbidity and can provide a survival benefit. Careful preoperative planning and choice of conduit require special attention for this operation, and expertise from other surgical services may be needed for assistance with the resection or reconstruction. The ability to perform an R0 resection is of utmost importance, and resection should not be undertaken if this is not considered feasible at the outset. As the trend toward multimodality therapy for EC permeates the medical community, an increasing number of patients with esophageal carcinoma are presenting with local-regional relapse after dCRT. It is important for the esophageal surgeon to be involved with the evaluation and treatment planning of these patients and offer salvage resection to appropriate candidates. The authors have shown that carefully selected patients undergoing a salvage resection can have outcomes similar to those undergoing a planned esophagectomy after CRT.

SUPPLEMENTARY DATA

Supplementary data related to this article are found online at http://dx.doi.org/10.1016/j.thorsurg.2013.08.001.

REFERENCES

1. Bedenne L, Michel P, Bouché O, et al. Chemoradiation followed by surgery compared with chemoradiation alone in squamous cancer of the esophagus. J Clin Oncol 2007;25(10):1160–8.
2. Stahl M, Stuschke M, Lehmann N, et al. Chemoradiation with and without surgery in patients with locally advanced squamous cell carcinoma of the esophagus. J Clin Oncol 2005;23(10):2310–7.
3. Borghesi S, Hawkins MA, Tait D. Oesophagectomy after definitive chemoradiation in patients with locally advanced oesophageal cancer. Clin Oncol (R Coll Radiol) 2008;20:221–6.
4. Morita M, Kumashiro R, Hisamatsu Y, et al. Clinical significance of salvage esophagectomy for remnant or recurrent cancer following definitive chemoradiotherapy. J Gastroenterol 2011;46:1284–91.
5. Gardner-Thorpe J, Hardwick R, Dwerryhouse S. Salvage oesophagectomy after local failure of definitive chemoradiation. Br J Surg 2007;94:1059–66.
6. Nishimura M, Daiko H, Yoshida J, et al. Salvage esophagectomy following definitive chemoradiotherapy. Gen Thorac Cardiovasc Surg 2007;55:461–5.
7. Tachimori Y, Kanamori N, Uemura N, et al. Salvage esophagectomy after high-dose chemoradiotherapy for esophageal squamous cell carcinoma. J Thorac Cardiovasc Surg 2009;137:49–54.
8. Marks J, Hofstetter W, Correa A, et al. Salvage esophagectomy after failed definitive chemoradiation for esophageal adenocarcinoma. Ann Thorac Surg 2012;94(4):1126–33.
9. Swisher S, Wynn P, Putnam J, et al. Salvage esophagectomy for recurrent tumors after definitive chemotherapy and radiotherapy. J Thorac Cardiovasc Surg 2002;123(1):175–8.
10. Ascioti A, Hofstetter W, Miller M, et al. Long-segment, supercharged, pedicled jejunal flap for

total esophageal reconstruction. J Thorac Cardiovasc Surg 2005;130(5):1391–8.

11. Swisher S, Hofstetter W, Miller M. The supercharged microvascular jejunal interposition. Semin Thorac Cardiovasc Surg 2007;19(1):56–65.

12. Kawauchi Y, Fu K, Morimoto T, et al. Aortoesophageal fistula after radiation therapy for esophageal cancer (with video). Gastrointest Endosc 2011;74(4):922.

13. Isasti G, Olallab E, Gómez-Doblasa J. Aortoesophageal fistula: an uncommon complication after stent-graft repair of an aortic thoracic aneurysm. Interact Cardiovasc Thorac Surg 2009;9(4):683–4.

14. Ghosh SK, Rahman FZ, Bown S, et al. Survival following treatment of aortoesophageal fistula with dual esophageal and aortic intervention. Case Rep Gastroenterol 2011;5(1):40–4.

15. Morita M, Nakanoko T, Kubo N, et al. Two-Stage operation for high-risk Patients with thoracic esophageal cancer: an old operation revisited. Ann Surg Oncol 2011;18:2613–21.

16. Sugimachi K, Kitamura M, Maekawa S, et al. Two stage operation for poor-risk patients with carcinoma of the esophagus. J Surg Oncol 1987; 36(2):105–9.

17. Bhat M, Dar M, Lone G, et al. Use of pedicled omentum in esophagogastric anastomosis for prevention of anastomotic leak. Ann Thorac Surg 2006;82(5): 1857–62.

18. Dai J, Zhang Z, Min J, et al. Wrapping of the omental pedicle flap around esophagogastric anastomosis after esophagectomy for esophageal cancer. Surgery 2011;149(3):404–10.

19. Sepesi B, Swisher S, Walsh G, et al. Omental reinforcement of the thoracic esophago-gastric anastomosis. Presented at 2012 AATS.

20. Low D, Kunz S, Schembre D, et al. Esophagectomy–it's not just about mortality anymore: standardized perioperative clinical pathways improve outcomes in patients with esophageal cancer. J Gastrointest Surg 2007;11(11):1395–402.

Quality of Life in Patients with Esophageal Cancer

Gail E. Darling, MD, FRCSC

KEYWORDS

- Esophageal cancer • Health-related quality of life • Dysphagia • Esophagectomy • EORTC QLQ-30
- OES-18 • FACT-E • Palliation

KEY POINTS

- Patient perception of health-related quality of life (HRQOL) is the outcome of interest, not that of the health care professional, family, or caregiver.
- HRQOL is more than a list of symptoms, and although symptoms of the disease or treatment may affect HRQOL, other factors contribute and may be even more important.
- HRQOL assessed in longterm followup after esophagectomy is similar to the normal population.
- HRQOL assessed in early follow-up of patients treated with definitive chemoradiation may be better than in patients treated with surgery alone or chemoradiation followed by surgery, but survival may be superior in patients whose treatment includes surgery.
- HRQOL recovers more quickly after minimally invasive surgery or transhiatal esophagectomy than after open esophagectomy.

INTRODUCTION

Esophageal cancer has a significant effect on quality of life (QOL). Most patients present for medical attention because of dysphagia. Although dysphagia is just one symptom of esophageal cancer, it has a significant adverse effect on QOL, not just because of the physical problem of difficulty swallowing or the weight loss that may result, but because sharing a meal with friends or family is a social event, and inability to swallow comfortably or regurgitation of food may lead to withdrawal from social situations and isolation. Sadness or depression may result irrespective of the cancer prognosis.

Evaluating outcomes of cancer therapy has primarily focused on effectiveness in terms of survival, the side effects of treatment, and treatment-related mortality. It is only in the past decade or so that health-related quality of life (HRQOL) has been recognized as an important outcome measure of therapy for esophageal cancer, particularly because of the low rate of cure in esophageal cancer despite aggressive therapies. For many patients, cure of their cancer may make toxicity of treatment acceptable, but the investment of time and the side effects of treatment may be less acceptable if the cancer is not cured.

It is the patient's perspective that is most important in assessing QOL, not the perception of the spouse, family, friend, or health care professional. Therefore, HRQOL questions must be answered by the patient, and many HRQOL instruments are self-administered. HRQOL assessment evaluates how the patient's health state affects their QOL. Although symptoms may adversely impact QOL, HRQOL is not just a list of symptoms (either of the disease or its treatment), but also evaluates various domains, including physical aspects of function, social functioning, emotional well-being, and functional abilities. This article focuses on the assessment of HRQOL in patients with esophageal cancer after both curative- and palliative-intent therapy.

Division of Thoracic Surgery, Department of Surgery, Toronto General Hospital, University Health Network, University of Toronto, 200 Elizabeth Street, 9N-955, Toronto, Ontario M5G 2C4, Canada
E-mail address: gail.darling@uhn.ca

Thorac Surg Clin 23 (2013) 569–575
http://dx.doi.org/10.1016/j.thorsurg.2013.07.011
1547-4127/13/$ – see front matter © 2013 Elsevier Inc. All rights reserved.

HRQOL INSTRUMENTS

QOL instruments include generic and disease-specific instruments. The Medical Outcomes Study 36 Item Short Form Health Survey (MOS SF-36) has been used to assess HRQOL across a broad range of diseases and conditions.[1,2] This instrument is useful in comparing HRQOL in a population of patients with a specific disease relative to the general population, or comparing HRQOL in patients with different health conditions. The MOS SF-36 assesses 8 health domains (physical function, role physical, pain, general health perception, energy/vitality, social functioning, role emotional, and mental health) and provides 2 summary measures of physical and mental well-being.

Disease-specific HRQOL instruments are used for specific disease states. In esophageal cancer, the most common instrument used is the European Organization for Research and Treatment of Cancer (EORTC) QLQ (quality of life questionnaire)-30 with the esophageal cancer disease-specific module OES (oesophageal)-18 (previously the OES-24). Using a 4-point Likert scale, the EORTC QLQ-30 includes 5 functional scales (physical function, emotional function, social function, cognitive function, and role function) and 3 symptom scales (fatigue, nausea, and pain). There are 6 single-item questions (regarding dyspnea, insomnia, appetite, constipation, diarrhea, and financial worries), which are also evaluated using a 4-point Likert scale. Global QOL is assessed by a single question using a 7-point Likert scale. The esophageal module (OES-18) includes 18 items addressing areas such as dysphagia, swallowing, choking, eating, reflux, taste, abdominal pain, odynophagia, dry mouth, cough, and voice difficulties. The OG (oesophageal-gastric)-25 is a similar instrument devised for esophagogastric tumors.[3,4]

The Functional Assessment of Cancer Therapy-General (FACT-G) may be used to evaluate HRQOL for any cancer and consists of 28 questions covering the domains of physical well-being, functional well-being, social well-being, and emotional well-being using a 5-point Likert scale. A major difference between the FACT-G and the EORTC QLQ-30 is the assessment of global HRQOL, which is evaluated by a single question in the EORTC QLQ-30, whereas the FACT-G uses a summation of the 4 subscales to generate a global QOL score.[5] A disease-specific module is added for esophageal cancer, which consists of 17 items addressing areas such as eating, swallowing, enjoyment of food, voice, dry mouth, appetite, cough, choking, and pain, each evaluated using a 5-point Likert scale to generate a summary score of esophageal-specific concerns.[6]

In addition to these QOL instruments, several other instruments have been used to evaluate HRQOL in esophageal cancer, including the Rotterdam Symptom Checklist, Spitzer Quality of Life Index, Profile of Mood States, Gastrointestinal Quality of Life Index, and the University of Washington Quality of Life Scale.[7]

HRQOL AFTER CURATIVE-INTENT TREATMENT FOR ESOPHAGEAL CANCER
Long-term Effect of Esophagectomy on HRQOL

A systematic review of HRQOL assessed using the EORTC QLQ-30 or MOS SF-36 after esophagectomy found 21 studies, 5 of which used the MOS SF-36 and 16 used the EORTC QLQ-30; 14 of 16 also used the OES-18. Five studies compared patients who underwent esophagectomy with healthy subjects using the MOS SF-36 at follow-up intervals of 3 to 5 years. These studies found that with respect to pain and mental health, patients who underwent esophagectomy had significantly better scores generally than the healthy population but significantly poorer HRQOL with respect to physical function, vitality, and health perception. Work, activities of daily living, and emotional and social function were similar to the healthy population.[8] However, these 5 studies included patients with cancer and those with high-grade dysplasia, some resected with transhiatal esophagectomy and some with transthoracic esophagectomy. Conceptually it seems that this heterogeneity of the patient population would likely impact the HRQOL scores at least for physical and functional domains.[9,10] In a study of only patients with high-grade dysplasia, physical and emotional scores were similar or better than those for age-matched controls.[11] Comparing 5-year survivors after esophagectomy with age- and sex-matched nonpatient controls using the EORTC QLQ-30 and the OES-18, Derogar and Lagergren[12] reported that global HRQOL had stabilized or improved in 83% of patients by 6 months postoperatively, and these findings persisted to 5 years postoperatively. Similarly, physical function was stable or improved in 86% of patients from 6 months to 5 years postoperatively, and scores were similar to those of the nonpatient population. However, these authors found a subgroup of patients (14%) in whom HRQOL deteriorated over time even though their 6-month scores were not significantly different from those of patients whose HRQOL was stable or improved over time. Patients in whom HRQOL deteriorated over time had more symptoms and worse function in all domains. It seems unusual that this group would have such globally poor function and worse symptoms at 5 years, even though their 6-month scores were similar to those of the groups whose HRQOL improved or was stable. This finding may be from what is termed *response shift*, wherein the patient's perception of their QOL changes because of changes in their own values, priorities, or interpretation of QOL.

HRQOL as a Predictive Tool

Poor HRQOL scores at 6 months postoperatively (categorized as good vs poor function or minor/no symptoms vs symptomatic) were found to be predictive of survival, with poor function and symptoms predicting increased mortality **Table 1**.[13] Poor HRQOL scores before treatment also suggest worse survival.[14]

Safieddine and colleagues[15] found that patients who developed recurrence and died within 12 months of surgery experienced declining HRQOL postoperatively, which did not recover by 3 months even before recurrent cancer had been detected through imaging or clinical assessment, whereas patients who survived more than 1 year postoperatively had overall HRQOL scores that improved postoperatively and continued to improve beyond 3 months to 1 year after surgery **Fig. 1**. Blazeby and colleagues[16] also found that HRQOL continued to improve above baseline in patients who survived more than 1 year. In particular, Djarv and colleagues[14] reported that recovery of physical function postoperatively was associated with improved survival.

Early Postoperative HRQOL

Surgery clearly has a negative impact on HRQOL in the early postoperative period. Using the EORTC

Table 1
HRQOL at 6 months predicts decreased survival

HRQOL Domain	Hazard Ratio	95% Confidence Interval
Global HRQL	1.55	1.19–2.02
Physical function	1.56	1.23–1.99
Social function	1.52	1.19–1.94
Fatigue	1.65	1.30–2.11
Pain	1.45	1.22–1.87
Dyspnea	1.54	1.19–2.01
Appetite loss	1.69	1.32–2.14
Dysphagia	1.69	1.13–2.51
Esophageal pain	1.29	1.02–1.65

Data from Djarv T, Lagergren P. Six-month post-operative quality of life predicts long term survival after oesophageal cancer. Eur J Cancer 2011;47:530–5.

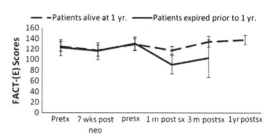

Fig. 1. Mean FACT-E scores in patients treated with chemoradiation and esophagectomy. Overall mean FACT-E scores decline during and after chemoradiation but recover to baseline levels before surgery. After esophagectomy, overall mean FACT-E scores again decline but, in patients who survive at least 12 months postesophagectomy, begin to recover by 1 month postoperatively and then continue to increase and are above baseline levels by 12 months postoperatively. In contrast, patients who die of recurrent cancer within 12 months of surgery have more decline in overall FACT-E scores postoperatively, which never recover to baseline levels even at 3 months postoperatively, even before recurrence is suspected or evident through clinical evaluation or imaging. Postsx, postesophagectomy; post neo, post neoadjuvant chemoradiation; presx, before surgery, approximately 6 to 8 weeks after completion of neoadjuvant chemoradiation; pretx, before treatment/baseline. (*From* Safieddine N, Xu W, Quadri SM, et al. Health related quality of life in esophageal cancer: effect of neoadjuvant chemoradiotherapy followed by surgical intervention. J Thorac Cardiovasc Surg 2009;137:39; with permission.)

QLQ-30, essentially all aspects of HRQOL are significantly worse when measured at 6 weeks postoperatively. By 6 to 9 months, overall HRQOL and the domains of emotional, role functional, and social function recover to baseline.[16,17] Brooks and colleagues[18] reported similar results using the FACT-Esophageal (FACT-E). Safieddine and colleagues[15] reported somewhat different results. Total FACT-E scores, physical well-being, and functional well-being scores declined significantly after surgery, but emotional and social well-being scores remained stable postoperatively throughout trimodality (chemoradiation and surgery) treatment. Also, overall HRQOL recovered to baseline levels by 3 months after surgery. Only physical well-being remained significantly below baseline levels at 3 months.

Effect of Preoperative Chemoradiation on HRQOL After Esophagectomy

Some investigators have suggested that preoperative chemoradiation has a profound adverse effect on HRQOL, with patients never recovering their baseline HRQOL.[8] However, studies using both the EORTC QLQ-30 and OES-18 and the FACT-E report that although HRQOL decreases significantly during chemoradiation, scores recover to baseline levels before and after surgery Fig. 2.[15,17]

When comparing HRQOL in patients treated with surgery alone versus those treated with chemoradiation followed by surgery, conflicting results are reported. Blazeby and colleagues[17] found no adverse impact on recovery of HRQOL postoperatively in patients treated with preoperative chemotherapy or chemoradiation compared with those treated with surgery alone. Hurmuzlu and colleagues,[19] however, found that patients treated with trimodality therapy had worse HRQOL than those treated with surgery alone when assessed approximately 1 year postoperatively. Both groups used the EORTC QLQ-30 and OES-18; however, patients in the Norwegian study[19] received high-dose radiation to 66 Gy with concomitant cisplatin (100 mg/m^2) and 5-fluorouracil (1000 mg/m^2), whereas in the British study,[17] patients were treated with a lower dose of both cisplatin (60 mg/m^2) and 5-fluorouracil (300 mg/m^2) and a total radiation dose of 45 Gy. This discrepancy illustrates one of the difficulties in assessing the results of treatment for esophageal cancer: not only do surgical approaches differ and have differing effects on HRQOL, but chemotherapy and radiation therapy regimens differ. These differences may explain the contradictory conclusions of the Norwegian and British studies, highlighting the importance of assessing HRQOL when evaluating different treatment regimens. Worse HRQOL would support using a less-toxic regimen, unless significant improvement in survival is seen.

Effect of Surgery Versus Definitive Chemoradiation on HRQOL

Several nonrandomized studies have compared definitive chemoradiation versus surgery either alone or after neoadjuvant chemoradiation,[7] reporting worse HRQOL in patients undergoing surgery. One study found that the only independent predictor of global HRQOL was esophageal preservation.[20] However, a randomized trial of surgery alone compared with definitive chemoradiation for operable squamous cell cancer of the esophagus reported no difference in HRQOL between the groups in terms of overall HRQOL or functional or symptom subscales at any time point. No difference was seen in baseline scores between the groups, and survival was similar. In evaluating longitudinal scores, patients who underwent surgery experienced worsened physical function up to 6 months postoperatively, whereas physical function was at its worst 3 months after chemoradiation.[21]

Effect of Surgical Technique on HRQOL

Confounding factors in evaluating HRQOL after esophagectomy include variability in baseline HRQOL, the use of preoperative chemotherapy or chemoradiation, different surgical techniques, and postoperative complications. Comparing transhiatal with transthoracic esophagectomy, de Boer and colleagues[10] found that HRQOL was similar for both approaches, except that patients

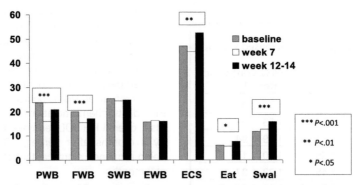

Fig. 2. FACT-E scores in patients with esophageal cancer treated with preoperative chemoradiation. Emotional well-being (EWB) and social well-being (SWB) are stable from baseline through chemoradiotherapy to preoperative assessment. Physical well-being (PWB) and functional well-being (FWB) decline significantly during chemoradiation but recover by 12 to 14 weeks, which is just before surgery. Differences between baseline and preoperative values are not statistically significant. The esophageal cancer subscale (ECS) and the eating (eat) and swallowing (swal) subscales improve significantly from baseline to preoperative assessment. (*Data from* Safieddine N, Xu W, Quadri SM, et al. Health related quality of life in esophageal cancer: effect of neoadjuvant chemoradiotherapy followed by surgical intervention. J Thorac Cardiovasc Surg 2009;137:36–42.)

who had a transhiatal esophagectomy had fewer symptoms and were more active at 3 months after surgery. Not surprisingly, in comparing transhiatal, transthoracic, and minimally invasive esophagectomy at 1 year postoperatively, no differences were seen in global HRQOL of any of the functional scales, single items, or symptoms scales of the EORTC QLQ-30 and OES-18.[22] When HRQOL was compared at 1 to 3 months after surgery, however, significant differences were seen between open and minimally invasive esophagectomy in terms of role functioning and pain.[23] Comparing patients undergoing a minimally invasive esophagectomy versus the normal population using the MOS SF-36, Luketich and colleagues[24] reported no difference in terms of physical or mental scores or overall global QOL measured at a mean of 19 months (range, 1–68 months) postoperatively.

Esophagectomy alone or after chemoradiation leads to decreased HRQOL, which is at its lowest point approximately 6 weeks postoperatively. HRQOL gradually improves over time, returning to baseline levels by 3 to 6 months. Although overall HRQOL returns to baseline, many patients still have significant symptoms at 3 to 6 months postoperatively, and these symptoms may persist for many months. Therefore, physical function or well-being often remains below baseline even at 9 to 12 months postoperatively.[7,15]

Complications after esophagectomy are common, and major complications contribute to worse HRQOL in the long term as assessed by symptom scores, particularly with respect to dyspnea, fatigue, poor appetite, choking, reflux, and esophageal pain. However, in terms of patient perception of global QOL, no significant difference was seen between those who experienced no complications and those experiencing at least one major complication, illustrating that symptoms do not necessarily correlate with patient perception of QOL.[25]

Using HRQOL to Evaluate Outcomes of Treatment in Esophageal Cancer

Although the use of HRQOL as an outcome measure of interest in esophageal cancer is an important advance in the management of patients with esophageal cancer, many confounding factors clearly affect the results of these studies. Significant variability exists among patients, stages of disease, surgical approaches, and chemotherapy or chemoradiation regimens. This variability may explain contradictory results in the published literature.

When HRQOL is compared before and after treatment, the effect of the treatment may be assessed. A disease-specific measure is most appropriate in this situation; however, the use of patient baseline data may be problematic, because HRQOL may be variable among patients and is also affected by tumor factors. When comparing patients with and without esophageal cancer, a generic instrument such as the MOS SF-36 is appropriate. But which instrument is most appropriate in longitudinal studies? The answer depends on the purpose of the study. In evaluating recovery after treatment, a disease-specific instrument may be appropriate, but if one wants to know when the patient who has been treated for esophageal cancer recovers to the population "norm," a generic instrument should be used. An important confounding factor may be that the patient's perception of their QOL may evolve over time as their expectations, values, or priorities shift.[25]

In authors reporting HRQOL in the literature, a tendency exists to report the global HRQOL. In the EORTC QLQ-30, this is the result of a single question evaluated on a 7-item Likert scale, whereas in the FACT-G, the global HRQOL is derived from the sum of the 4 domains of physical well-being, functional well-being, emotional well-being, and social well-being. Which approach provides a more valid reflection of the patient's perception?

The use of global HRQOL may reduce the utility of the HRQOL instruments. The use of the subscales may provide important information that is not apparent from the global HRQOL assessment. As has been demonstrated in patients with esophageal cancer postesophagectomy, physical function and symptom scores remain abnormal more than 6 months postoperatively, yet social, functional, and emotional well-being are at or above baseline.

HRQOL After Palliative Intent Treatment for Esophageal Cancer

Palliation of dysphagia is a primary goal of all esophageal cancer therapy. When curative intent therapy is inappropriate, available treatment options for palliation of dysphagia include esophageal stenting, external-beam radiation, brachytherapy, neodymium:yttrium-aluminum-garnet laser; photodynamic therapy, thermoablative therapy, and chemotherapy. The ideal treatment would provide immediate and durable relief of dysphagia without the need for reintervention.

The most common methods for palliation of dysphagia are external-beam radiation, brachytherapy, and self-expanding metals stents (SEMS). SEMS have largely replaced previous

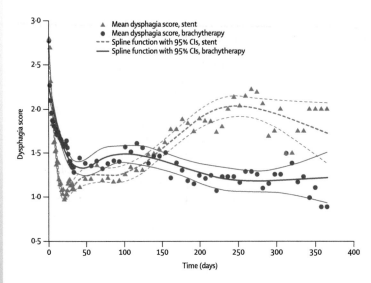

Fig. 3. Comparison of SEMS and brachytherapy in palliation of dysphagia in esophageal cancer. Although SEMS provide almost immediate improvement in dysphagia, over time dysphagia scores worsen. In patients treated with brachytherapy, dysphagia scores improved more slowly, but improvement was more durable over time. Overall HRQOL scores also worsened over time in patients with SEMS, but were maintained in the brachytherapy group (data not shown). (*From* Homs MY, Steyerber EW, Eijkenboom WM, et al. Single-dose brachytherapy versus metal stent placement for the palliation of dysphagia from oesophageal cancer: multicentre randomised trial. Lancet 2004;364:1497–504; with permission.)

stents because of their ease of insertion, reduced rate of perforation, and reduced mortality. SEMS may be associated with reduced QOL in the first 6 weeks after insertion because of pain associated with insertion.[26] However, 2 randomized trials of SEMS versus brachytherapy reported that SEMS provided almost immediate relief of dysphagia, whereas brachytherapy was associated with more durable/stable relief of dysphagia and overall improved QOL **Fig. 3**.[27,28] Recurrent dysphagia and other delayed complications may occur in 30% to 45% of patients after SEMS placement because of tumor overgrowth, hemorrhage, stent migration, food bolus obstruction, and fistula formation. After brachytherapy, up to 15% of patients may have persistent dysphagia.[29] Durable improvement in dysphagia without the need for reintervention and reduced complications may account for the overall improved QOL in patients treated with brachytherapy compared with those treated with SEMS. Brachytherapy may be more appropriate for patients who may have more prolonged survival, whereas SEMS may be more appropriate for those with very limited survival.

SUMMARY

Assessment of HRQOL is an important outcome measure in evaluating treatment for esophageal cancer, whether for curative or palliative intent. Clinicians must realize that the patient's perception of their QOL is the most important consideration, and that HRQOL is not simply a list of symptoms. Assessment of HRQOL in esophageal cancer in the setting of curative-intent therapy is complicated by the variety of treatment approaches, including different surgical techniques, varying doses of radiation, and differing chemotherapy regimens. Variability in patient factors even at the time of baseline measurement may make comparisons difficult, and shifts in patient responses over time may confound the results of long-term studies. Despite these challenges, performing a HRQOL assessment provides the patient, caregiver, and health care provider with important information when comparing therapeutic options.

REFERENCES

1. McHorney CA, Ware JE Jr, Racek AE. The MOS 36-item Short-Form Health Survey (SF-36): II. Psychometric and clinical tests of validity in measuring physical and mental health constructs. Med Care 1993;31:247–63.
2. McHorney CA, Ware JE Jr, Lu JF, et al. The MOS 36 item Short-Form Health Survey (SF-36): III. Tests of data quality, scaling assumptions, and reliability across diverse patient groups. Med Care 1994;32:40–66.
3. Groenvold M, Klee MC, Sprangers MA, et al. Validation of the EORTC QLQ-30 quality of life questionnaire through combined qualitative and quantitative assessment of patient–observer agreement. J Clin Epidemiol 1997;50:441–50.
4. Blazeby JM, Conroy T, Hammerlid E, et al. Clinical and psychometric validation of an EORTC questionnaire module, the EORTC QLQ-OES18, to assess quality of life in patients with oesophageal cancer. Eur J Cancer 2003;39:1384–94.
5. Cella DF, Tulsky DS, Gray G, et al. The functional assessment of cancer therapy scale: development and validation of the general measure. J Clin Oncol 1993;11:570–9.

6. Darling G, Eton DT, Sulman J, et al. Validation of the functional assessment of cancer therapy esophageal cancer subscale. Cancer 2006;107:854–63.

7. Sanghera SS, Nurkin SJ, Demmy TL. Quality of life after an esophagectomy. Surg Clin North Am 2012; 92:1315–35.

8. Scarpa M, Valente S, Alferi R, et al. Systematic review of health-related quality of life after esophagectomy for esophageal cancer. World J Gastroenterol 2011;17:4660–74.

9. McLarty AJ, Deschamps C, Trastek VF, et al. Esophageal resection for cancer of the esophagus: long term function and quality of life. Ann Thorac Surg 1997;63:1568–72.

10. de Boer AG, van Lanschot JJ, van Sandick JW, et al. Quality of life after transhiatal compared with extended transthoracic resection for adenocarcinoma of the esophagus. J Clin Oncol 2004;22:4202–8.

11. Headrick JR, Nichols FC 3rd, Miller DL, et al. High grade esophageal dysplasia: long terms survival and quality of life after esophagectomy. Ann Thorac Surg 2002;73:1697–702.

12. Derogar M, Lagergren P. Health related quality of life among 5 year survivors of esophageal cancer surgery: a prospective population based study. J Clin Oncol 2012;30:413–8.

13. Djarv T, Lagergren P. Six-month post-operative quality of life predicts long term survival after oesophageal cancer. Eur J Cancer 2011;47:530–5.

14. Djarv T, Metcalfe C, Avery KN, et al. Prognostic value of changes in health related quality of life scores during curative treatment for esophagogastric cancer. J Clin Oncol 2010;10:1666–70.

15. Safieddine N, Xu W, Quadri SM, et al. Health related quality of life in esophageal cancer: effect of neoadjuvant chemoradiotherapy followed by surgical intervention. J Thorac Cardiovasc Surg 2009;137:36–42.

16. Blazeby JM, Farndon JR, Donovan J, et al. A prospective longitudinal study examining the quality of life of patients with esophageal carcinoma. Cancer 2000;88:1781–7.

17. Blazeby JM, Metcalfe C, Nicklin J, et al. Association between quality of life scores and short-term outcome after surgery for cancer of the oesophagus or gastric cardia. Br J Surg 2005;92:1502–7.

18. Brooks JA, Kesler KA, Johnson CS, et al. Prospective analysis of quality of life after surgical resection for esophageal cancer: preliminary results. J Surg Oncol 2002;81:185–94.

19. Hurmuzlu M, Aarstad HJ, Aarstad AK, et al. Health-related quality of life in longer-term survivors after high-dose chemoradiotherapy followed by surgery in esophageal cancer. Dis Esophagus 2011;24: 39–47.

20. Ariga H, Nemoto K, Miyazaki S, et al. Prospective comparison of surgery alone and chemoradiotherapy with selective surgery in resectable squamous cell carcinoma of the esophagus. Int J Radiat Oncol Biol Phys 2009;75:348–56.

21. Teoh AY, Chiu PW, Wong TC, et al. Functional performance and quality of life in patients with squamous esophageal carcinoma receiving surgery or chemoradiation. Ann Surg 2011;253:1–5.

22. Sundaram A, Geronimo JC, Willer BL, et al. Survival and quality of life after minimally invasive esophagectomy: a single surgeon experience. Surg Endosc 2012;26:168–76.

23. Nafteux P, Moons J, Coosemans W, et al. Minimally invasive oesophagectomy: a valuable alternative to open oesophagectomy for the treatment of early oesophageal and gastro-oesophageal junction carcinoma. Eur J Cardiothorac Surg 2011;40: 1455–65.

24. Luketich JD, Alvelo-Rivera M, Buenaventura PO, et al. Minimally invasive esophagectomy: outcomes in 222 patients. Ann Surg 2003;238:486–94.

25. Derogar M, Orsini N, Sadr-Azodi O, et al. Influence of major postoperative complications on health-related quality of life among long term survivors of esophageal cancer surgery. J Clin Oncol 2012;30: 1615–9.

26. Shenfine J, McNamee P, Steen N, et al. A randomized controlled clinical trial of palliative therapies for patients with inoperable esophageal cancer. Am J Gastroenterol 2009;104:1674–85.

27. Homs MY, Steyerber EW, Eijkenboom WM, et al. Single-dose brachytherapy versus metal stent placement for the palliation of dysphagia from oesophageal cancer: multicentre randomised trial. Lancet 2004;364:1497–504.

28. Bergquist H, Wenger U, Johnsson E, et al. Stent insertion of endoluminal brachytherapy as palliation of patients with advanced cancer of the esophagus and gastroesophageal junction. Results a randomized, controlled clinical trial. Dis Esophagus 2005; 18:131–9.

29. Homs MY, Kuipers EJ, Siersema PD. Palliative therapy. J Surg Oncol 2005;92:246–56.

Index

Note: Page numbers of article titles are in **boldface** type.

thoracic.theclinics.com

United States Postal Service

Statement of Ownership, Management, and Circulation
(All Periodicals Publications Except Requestor Publications)

1. Publication Title	2. Publication Number	3. Filing Date
Thoracic Surgery Clinics	0 1 3 - 1 2 6	9/14/13

4. Issue Frequency	5. Number of Issues Published Annually	6. Annual Subscription Price
Feb, May, Aug, Nov	4	$335.00

7. Complete Mailing Address of Known Office of Publication *(Not printer) (Street, city, county, state, and ZIP+4®)*

Elsevier Inc.
360 Park Avenue South
New York, NY 10010-1710

Contact Person
Stephen R. Bushing
Telephone (Include area code)
215-239-3688

8. Complete Mailing Address of Headquarters or General Business Office of Publisher *(Not printer)*

Elsevier Inc., 360 Park Avenue South, New York, NY 10010-1710

9. Full Names and Complete Mailing Addresses of Publisher, Editor, and Managing Editor *(Do not leave blank)*

Publisher *(Name and complete mailing address)*

Linda Belfus, Elsevier, Inc., 1600 John F. Kennedy Blvd. Suite 1800, Philadelphia, PA 19103-2899

Editor *(Name and complete mailing address)*

Jessica McCool, Elsevier, Inc., 1600 John F. Kennedy Blvd. Suite 1800, Philadelphia, PA 19103-2899

Managing Editor *(Name and complete mailing address)*

Barbara Cohen-Kligerman, Elsevier, Inc., 1600 John F. Kennedy Blvd. Suite 1800, Philadelphia, PA 19103-2899

10. Owner *(Do not leave blank. If the publication is owned by a corporation, give the name and address of the corporation immediately followed by the names and addresses of all stockholders owning or holding 1 percent or more of the total amount of stock. If not owned by a corporation, give the names and addresses of the individual owners. If owned by a partnership or other unincorporated firm, give its name and address as well as those of each individual owner. If the publication is published by a nonprofit organization, give its name and address.)*

Full Name	Complete Mailing Address
Wholly owned subsidiary of	1600 John F. Kennedy Blvd, Ste. 1800
Reed/Elsevier, US holdings	Philadelphia, PA 19103-2899

11. Known Bondholders, Mortgagees, and Other Security Holders Owning or Holding 1 Percent or More of Total Amount of Bonds, Mortgages, or Other Securities. If none, check box ☐ None

Full Name	Complete Mailing Address
N/A	

12. Tax Status *(For completion by nonprofit organizations authorized to mail at nonprofit rates) (Check one)*
The purpose, function, and nonprofit status of this organization and the exempt status for federal income tax purposes:
☐ Has Not Changed During Preceding 12 Months
☐ Has Changed During Preceding 12 Months *(Publisher must submit explanation of change with this statement)*

PS Form 3526, September 2007 (Page 1 of 3 (Instructions Page 3)) PSN 7530-01-000-9931 PRIVACY NOTICE: See our Privacy policy in www.usps.com

---

13. Publication Title	14. Issue Date for Circulation Data Below
Thoracic Surgery Clinics	August 2013

15. Extent and Nature of Circulation			Average No. Copies Each Issue During Preceding 12 Months	No. Copies of Single Issue Published Nearest to Filing Date
a. Total Number of Copies *(Net press run)*			756	702
b. Paid Circulation (By Mail and Outside the Mail)	(1)	Mailed Outside-County Paid Subscriptions Stated on PS Form 3541. *(Include paid distribution above nominal rate, advertiser's proof copies, and exchange copies)*	402	360
	(2)	Mailed In-County Paid Subscriptions Stated on PS Form 3541 *(Include paid distribution above nominal rate, advertiser's proof copies, and exchange copies)*		
	(3)	Paid Distribution Outside the Mails Including Sales Through Dealers and Carriers, Street Vendors, Counter Sales, and Other Paid Distribution Outside USPS®	152	153
	(4)	Paid Distribution by Other Classes Mailed Through the USPS (e.g. First-Class Mail®)		
c. Total Paid Distribution *(Sum of 15b (1), (2), (3), and (4))*		▲	554	513
d. Free or Nominal Rate Distribution (By Mail and Outside the Mail)	(1)	Free or Nominal Rate Outside-County Copies Included on PS Form 3541	53	49
	(2)	Free or Nominal Rate In-County Copies Included on PS Form 3541		
	(3)	Free or Nominal Rate Copies Mailed at Other Classes Through the USPS (e.g. First-Class Mail)		
	(4)	Free or Nominal Rate Distribution Outside the Mail (Carriers or other means)		
e. Total Free or Nominal Rate Distribution (Sum of 15d (1), (2), (3) and (4))		▲	53	49
f. Total Distribution (Sum of 15c and 15e)		▲	607	562
g. Copies not Distributed *(See instructions to publishers #4 (page #3))*		▲	149	140
h. Total (Sum of 15f and g)		▲	756	702
i. Percent Paid (15c divided by 15f times 100)			91.27%	91.28%

16. Publication of Statement of Ownership
☐ If the publication is a general publication, publication of this statement is required. Will be printed ☐ Publication not required
in the November 2013 issue of this publication.

17. Signature and Title of Editor, Publisher, Business Manager, or Owner	Date
[signature] Stephen R. Bushing –Inventory/Distribution Coordinator	September 14, 2013

I certify that all information furnished on this form is true and complete. I understand that anyone who furnishes false or misleading information on this form or who omits material or information requested on the form may be subject to criminal sanctions (including fines and imprisonment) and/or civil sanctions (including civil penalties).

PS Form 3526, September 2007 (Page 2 of 3)

Moving?

Make sure your subscription moves with you!

To notify us of your new address, find your **Clinics Account Number** (located on your mailing label above your name), and contact customer service at:

Email: journalscustomerservice-usa@elsevier.com

800-654-2452 (subscribers in the U.S. & Canada)
314-447-8871 (subscribers outside of the U.S. & Canada)

Fax number: 314-447-8029

Elsevier Health Sciences Division
Subscription Customer Service
3251 Riverport Lane
Maryland Heights, MO 63043

*To ensure uninterrupted delivery of your subscription, please notify us at least 4 weeks in advance of move.

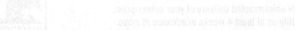

Printed and bound by CPI Group (UK) Ltd, Croydon, CR0 4YY

03/10/2024

01040309-0009